Contents

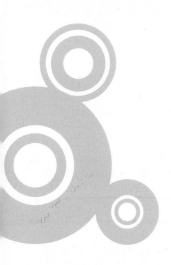

Introduction

This book has been written to help you achieve your Entry 3 and Level 1 qualification(s) in An introduction to the hair and beauty sector. It has been designed to provide you with all the information you need to guide you through the qualification for the main awarding bodies (City & Guilds, VTCT and Edexcel). It contains lots of technical information and real-life salon situations, including step-by-step photographs and illustrations of hairdressing and beauty therapy tasks. Some of the units are just about hairdressing, some are just about beauty therapy and some units relate to both (these are known as generic units).

Generic units

- Introduction to the hair and beauty sector (Entry 3 and Level 1)
- Follow health and safety in the salon (Level 1)
- Presenting a professional image in a salon (Entry 3 and Level 1)
- Salon reception duties (Level 1)
- Create an image using colour (Entry 3)

Hairdressing

- Shampoo and conditioning (Entry 3)
- Styling women's and men's hair (Level 1)
- Plaiting and twisting hair (Level 1)
- The art of dressing hair (Level 2)

Beauty therapy

- Skin care (Entry 3)
- Hand and foot care (Entry 3)
- Basic make-up application (Level 1)
- Themed face painting (Level 1)
- Nail art (Level 1)

Anatomy and physiology is covered in a separate unit but includes all of the hairdressing and beauty therapy information you will need.

This qualification is for anyone, at any age, who wishes to follow a career in either hairdressing or beauty therapy. The qualification acts as a good introduction to working in hairdressing or beauty therapy. You can begin to develop the necessary skills without having to show occupational competence, as is necessary when completing an NVQ qualification.

This qualification aims to provide you with:
- knowledge and skills (for Hairdressing or Beauty Therapy) that will provide a good foundation for further learning
- the skills to perform your own services and to assist colleagues in the salon
- an introduction to the hairdressing and beauty therapy industries and the skills required to work in them, helping you to decide whether this is the right career for you
- a chance to decide if you have the right personal skills to work in hairdressing and/or beauty therapy
- a general insight into the world of work.

Methods of assessment

While working towards this qualification, you will be assessed in a number of different ways, depending on the awarding body qualification you are taking:

City & Guilds

For City & Guilds, each assignment is divided into a series of tasks. To achieve each unit you have to complete all the tasks. For each unit there is likely to be:
- a task that requires you to prove your subject knowledge
- a task that requires you to find out and report on hairdressing and beauty treatments, products and fashions within the industry
- a task that requires you to show your practical skills.

VTCT

The method by which you are assessed will vary from unit to unit so you will need to check your record of assessment book for the specific requirements for each unit. For each of the practical units you will have a practical observation. You may also be questioned using oral questioning by your tutor or assessor to check your knowledge and understanding of the unit.

You will also need to produce a portfolio of evidence, either electronically or paper-based, to show your knowledge, understanding and skills. Your tutor or assessor will be able to give you further details on how to put it together and what it needs to contain.

Edexcel

Evidence will be assessed in a variety of ways. Your tutor or assessor will carry out observations of your practical skills. You will also have to complete some written assignments to test your knowledge and understanding. You will also be required to answer oral questions and have discussions with your tutor or assessor to demonstrate your understanding.

Features of this book

As you read through this book, you will notice several special features.
- Starter questions – an interesting question to start you thinking about the topic.
- Key terms – some of the words used in this book might be new to you, especially if they are **technical**. They appear in bold and the meaning of the word can be found in the margin, just as in the example given here.
- Top tips – bits of information and great pieces of advice that will help you work professionally.
- In the salon – an example of a real-life situation from a salon with questions to get you thinking about what you might have done in the same situation.
- Try it out – fun activities or tasks that get you to think about or build on what you have read.
- Just checking – questions at the end of each spread so you can make sure you have understood and remembered what you have learned so far.
- Functional skills icons – to help you spot activities that support functional skills. If you are taking this qualification as part of a foundation learning programme, you will attend classes on functional skills, English, Mathematics and ICT.

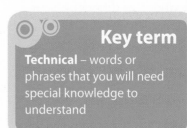

Key term

Technical – words or phrases that you will need special knowledge to understand

Introduction to the hair and beauty sector

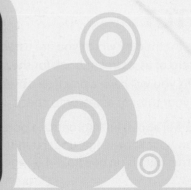

In this unit you will learn about:

- Working in the hairdressing and beauty industry
- Career opportunities and working patterns in the beauty and hairdressing sectors
- Different types of salon
- The main hairdressing services and beauty treatments available

Introduction

This is a very exciting time in your career as a hairdresser or beauty therapist. When you start out in this industry you have many choices. The hair and beauty sector provides many different **career opportunities** and a variety of **occupational roles**. Most of them offer different **working patterns** that can easily fit into your personal life. As you step into the hair and beauty sector you may already know where you want your career to take you. However, you may move into an area that you never thought about, as other opportunities arise.

Top tip

Because of the variety of jobs available in hair and beauty, try to train in different areas before you make your mind up what career path to follow. Don't limit yourself to only one thing – try a few and see where it takes you!

Key terms

Career opportunities – the types of places you may go to work as a hairdresser or beauty therapist; for example, salon, nail bar, health and fitness club

Occupational roles – the types of job you may carry out in your career; for example, salon manager, colour technician, make-up artist

Working patterns – the types of hours you work; for example, full-time, part-time, evenings only, days only

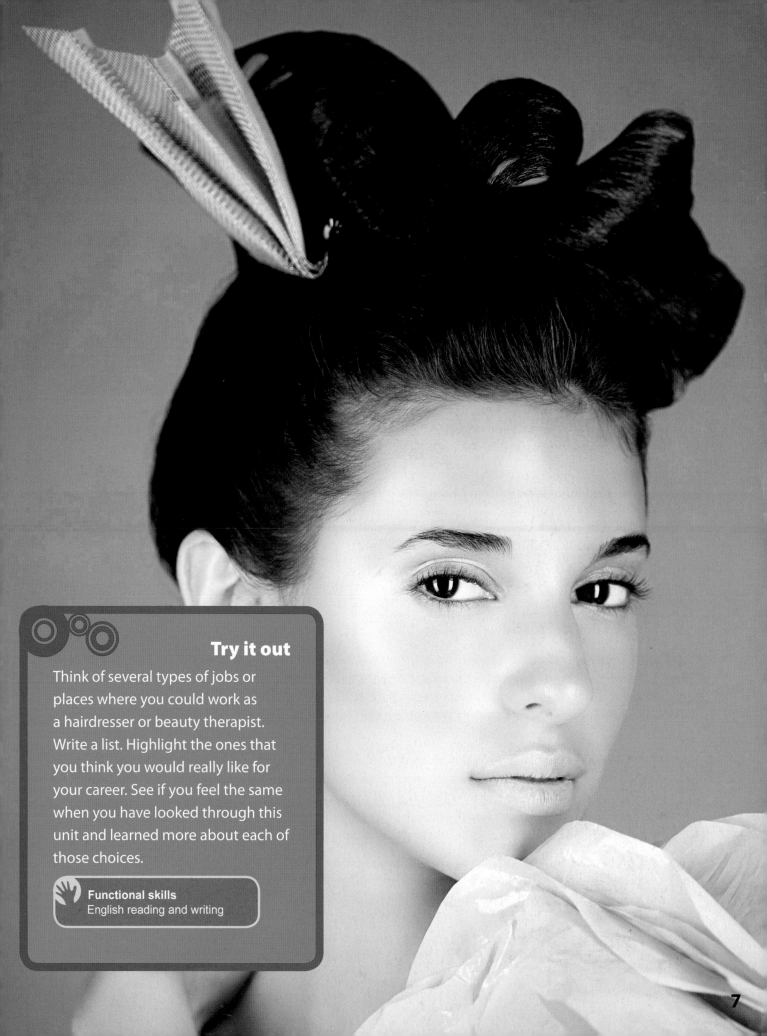

Try it out

Think of several types of jobs or places where you could work as a hairdresser or beauty therapist. Write a list. Highlight the ones that you think you would really like for your career. See if you feel the same when you have looked through this unit and learned more about each of those choices.

Functional skills
English reading and writing

Working in the hairdressing and beauty industry

In the salon – *Jignesh*

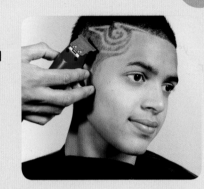

Jignesh began work as a junior in a barbers' shop, sweeping up and making drinks for clients and generally keeping the salon clean and tidy while the barbers were busy cutting hair. He watched and learned all the techniques and practised at home on his friends and family. He was particularly interested in pattern work, where images are cut into men's short hair to create a variety of patterns and designs. He found he had a real flair for this and decided to make a career out of cutting hair by enrolling at college on a Barbering NVQ Level 2 course.

While completing his course he observed the ladies' hairdressing classes and was drawn into ladies' hair too. As he worked full-time in a salon he signed up for an apprenticeship course so he could achieve NVQ Levels 2 and 3. He also began entering competitions and his work became famous, leading him into TV and photographic work.

Now he is qualified in both ladies' and men's hair, he has opened his own very successful hairdressing salon. He is continuing his work in competitions as a National judge and has more TV work lined up!

In the salon – *Katie*

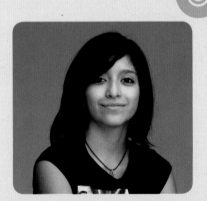

Katie began her hairdressing career straight from school at college on a full-time combined hair and beauty course. She studied for 3 years achieving NVQ Levels 1, 2 and 3 in Hairdressing and NVQ Levels 1 and 2 in Beauty Therapy. While a student she also entered competitions and greatly enjoyed her training.

When she had finished at college she decided to follow hairdressing instead of beauty and found herself a job in a city centre salon. Even though she enjoyed the work in the salon, she was always more interested in training the junior staff. Because of this, she decided to try assessing/teaching at the college where she originally trained.

After a few years, and having gained lots of experience teaching a variety of learners at college, she went to work as an educator at the Wella studios. Even though she only works for one product manufacturer, she is finding it extremely challenging and fulfilling. She is very satisfied in her chosen career.

In the salon – *Angela*

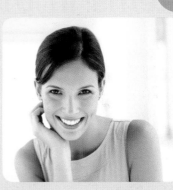

Angela studied Beauty Therapy at college on a full-time basis for 3 years and achieved NVQ Levels 2 and 3 in Beauty Therapy. Although she really loved Beauty, she felt that, at 21 years old, she couldn't be confined to working in a salon environment anymore. She wanted to travel and see some of the world. So she decided to combine the two and found a job working on a Steiner cruise liner as a beauty therapist.

Although the hours were often long, and she regularly worked 6 days a week, she loved the travelling. She also met some marvellous people. For 7 years she felt she had the perfect life but then, in her late twenties, she decided to leave the ships and return home to work. However, the routine of being based in a salon meant she was soon bored and she decided to begin teaching.

She now works as a full-time beauty therapy lecturer, working mainly with Level 3 and Level 4 learners and finds the variety this job offers much more stimulating.

In the salon – *Mykala*

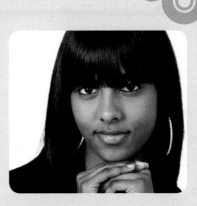

Mykala worked in a salon from the age of 14 as a Saturday junior. When she left school she carried on working there and attended college 1 day a week to gain her NVQs.

Mykala had a creative personality and was very interested in photographic and TV work, especially dramatic make-up. She went to night school and studied photographic and theatrical make-up, along with Beauty NVQ Level 2. This gave her all the qualifications she needed to find work within TV, theatre and photographic work. She looked for work in this area while continuing her job in the salon part-time.

However, she decided that she needed to work in this area full-time and left the salon to become a freelance TV and photographic stylist. Now she works up and down the country on different TV shows and on location wherever her job takes her. She has already built up a good reputation and is working on some high-profile shows.

Career opportunities and working patterns in the beauty sector

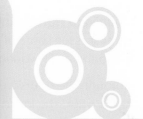

In this topic you will learn about:

- The occupational roles and career opportunities available in the beauty sector
- The working patterns in the beauty sector

Q **List all the different types of beauty therapy jobs you can think of. Do any of them appeal to you strongly?**

In the salon

Siobhain was working in the salon when an old college friend came in. Siobhain couldn't wait to tell her she was now the senior therapist and how well she had done for herself. Her friend then told her about her career on the cruise liners. She had earned plenty of money and was now a college lecturer with a good wage and holidays that fitted in with her young family. Siobhain found herself thinking, 'Why didn't I push myself to try something so exciting?'

Do you think her friend has chosen the most exciting career path, and if so, why? If not, why does Siobhain's job appeal more to you?

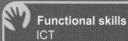

Try it out

Visit the website for Habia (Hair and Beauty Industry Authority) and the website for Connexions. Links to these sites have been made available at www.pearsonhotlinks.co.uk. Enter the express code P7511. Search for information about careers in beauty therapy. What is your dream career? How many different routes can you take?

 Functional skills
ICT

Top tip

All of the career options in beauty therapy can lead you to work with a variety of clients and earn different sums of money. Think carefully about what you want from a job in terms of personal satisfaction and reward.

Working patterns in the beauty sector

In beauty therapy, full-time work usually means working 40 hours per week and part-time work is anything less than this. Shift work involves working outside the hours of 9 am–5 pm, for example, 12 noon–8 pm. Most beauty therapists will have to work weekends – are you happy to do this for the rest of your working life? The following table shows the working patterns you may come across.

Type of job in beauty	Potential working pattern	Advantages and disadvantages
Therapist in a fitness centre	Shift work, full-time or part-time and weekends due to the long opening hours	Use of the gym facilities. Working shifts offers you more free time in the day. However, working late evenings and weekends may not be suitable.
Cruise liner therapist	Full-time, long days into early evenings and weekends	Travelling the world and meeting many different people. Working away from home for long periods of time.
Make-up artist, TV, theatre or photographic	Full-time or part-time, days, nights, weekends, no set place of work, travel involved	Flexible working where you may be able to choose your own working hours once you are established. Working long hours on shoots and travelling up and down the country can be time-consuming.
College lecturer	Full-time or part-time, days or evenings, term time only	May suit family commitments if you have children at school. Lots of work to do outside of college (preparation and marking, and college promotional events to attend).
Freelance therapist	Full-time or part-time, days or evenings	If you are successful and established you can choose your own working times to fit in around other commitments; for example, children. Clients will phone you evenings and weekends for appointments as you don't have set opening hours.

Just checking

1 If you achieve Level 3 Beauty Therapy, can you work for yourself visiting clients in their own homes?
2 Where can you find information about careers in beauty therapy?
3 What is the difference between working full-time or part-time?

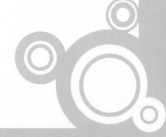

Career opportunities and working patterns in the hairdressing sector

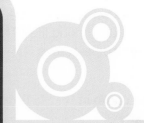

In this topic you will learn about:

- The occupational roles and career opportunities available in the hairdressing sector
- Working patterns in the hairdressing sector

With a partner, discuss the different areas of hairdressing you could work in. Does either of you already have a passion for a particular area?

In the salon

Paul had been working in a barbers' salon for the past 5 years and felt a little bored. One day a rep for a new product company came in to talk about their range. As it was quiet, Paul decided to listen and was **inspired** by the range and the possibilities it offered for a client's hair and **grooming routine**. The rep told him they needed salon trainers for their company and asked if he would be interested. Paul realised this was just the opportunity he needed to find his **passion** again in hairdressing. He contacted the company and after a successful interview he found himself driving around the country training and selling products. He loved his new job!

What do you think may have stopped Paul from progressing into this type of work before?

Try it out

Visit the website for Habia (Hair and Beauty Industry Authority) and the website for Connexions. Links to these sites have been made available at www.pearsonhotlinks.co.uk. Enter the express code P7511. Search for information about careers in hairdressing. What is your dream career? How many different routes can you take?

 Functional skills – ICT

Key terms

Inspired – finding interest in something, wanting to know more
Grooming routine – an expression used to describe a shaving or trimming routine for men's facial hair
Passion – enthusiastic, feeling strongly about something

Working patterns in the hairdressing sector

Hairdressing involves long days, most of which will be spent standing. It also involves working weekends. Do you think you can handle this long term as a career choice? The following table details the working patterns you may come across in a variety of hairdressing jobs.

Type of job in hairdressing	Potential working pattern	Advantages and disadvantages
Hairdressing in a fitness centre	Shift work, full-time or part-time and weekends due to the long opening hours	Use of the gym facilities. Working shifts offers you more free time in the day but working late evenings and weekends may not be suitable.
Cruise liner hairdresser	Full-time, long days into early evenings and weekends	Travelling the world and meeting many different people. Working away from home for long periods of time.
TV or theatre or photographic stylist	Full-time or part-time, days, nights, weekends	Flexible working where you may be able to choose your own working hours once you are established. Working long hours on shoots and travelling up and down the country can be time-consuming.
College lecturer	Full-time or part-time, days or evenings, term time only	May suit family commitments if you have children at school. Lots of work to do outside of college (preparation and marking, and college promotional events to attend).
Freelance hairdresser	Full-time or part-time, days or evenings	If you are successful and established you can choose your own working times to fit in around other commitments; for example, children. Clients will phone you evenings and weekends for appointments as you don't have set opening hours.

Just checking

1 If you achieve Level 3 Hairdressing, would you be qualified to work independently either as a salon owner or as a freelance hairdresser?
2 If you have problems standing for long periods because of injury or disability, would hairdressing be a good career choice for you?

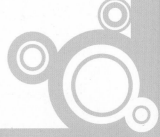

Different types of salon and the main hairdressing services and beauty treatments available

In this topic you will learn about:

- The different types of hair and beauty salons and the clients they attract
- The main hairdressing services and beauty treatments available in salons

Q Write down as many hairdressing services and beauty treatments as you can think of that a salon may offer. Pick up a price/treatment list from a local salon and compare it with your list to see what is available.

Types of salon and the clients they attract

The main hairdressing services offered in salons

Hairdressing service	Picture of service	Description of service
Cutting		Cutting hair either to restyle and create a new look or to trim off the ends
Setting		Using rollers or bendies to set the hair into curl or wave or just to add volume
Colouring		Changing hair colour, either temporary or more permanent, darker or lighter
Extensions		Adding extra hair to the natural hair using either human hair or synthetic hair
Patterning in hair		Using the razor and clippers to cut a pattern or design into very short hair

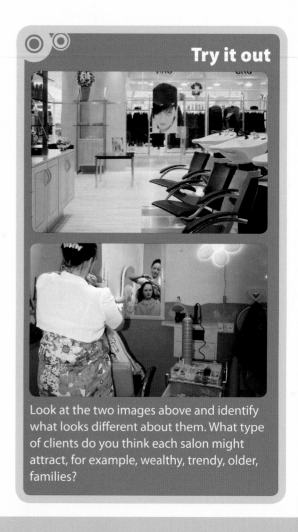

Try it out

Look at the two images above and identify what looks different about them. What type of clients do you think each salon might attract, for example, wealthy, trendy, older, families?

Main beauty treatments offered by salons

Type of service	Picture of service	Description of service
Manicure		A treatment on the hand and nails that softens the skin and tidies the nails before painting them
Waxing		Removal of hair using either hot or cold wax
Facials		A deep cleanse of the face using massage and masks to remove dirt and debris
Eyelash perming		Curling the lashes using a small cotton rod and lotions (lasts about 3 weeks)
Massage		A relaxing and comforting treatment where the hands are massaged using cream, oil or talc

Just checking

1 Do you think hairdressing and beauty services can be combined into one salon?

2 Below there is a list of salon names. Which do you think are hair salons and which are beauty salons?
   a A Cut Above the Rest
   b Body Perfect
   c The Style Inn
   d Aura Spa

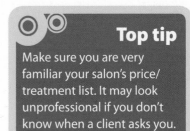

Top tip

Make sure you are very familiar your salon's price/treatment list. It may look unprofessional if you don't know when a client asks you.

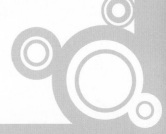

Follow health and safety in the salon

In this unit you will learn about:

- Hazards and risks in the salon
- The Health and Safety at Work Act
- COSHH (Control of Substances Hazardous to Health)
- PPE (Personal Protective Equipment)
- The Electricity at Work Regulations
- Safe manual handling
- Methods of sterilisation
- Emergencies and first aid
- Fire safety

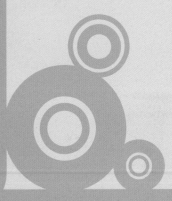

Introduction

There are lots of rules about health and safety in the salon. They are there to make sure that everyone is kept safe and free from harm.

This unit will help you to work safely in a salon by knowing what could possibly cause harm to you or someone else. It will also show you how to deal with these problems to make sure the salon is a safe place to work.

You will also learn what you should do if there is an accident or an emergency in the salon.

Top tip

Always follow the rules the salon owner gives you about working safely. This will make sure both you and the salon owner don't get into trouble.

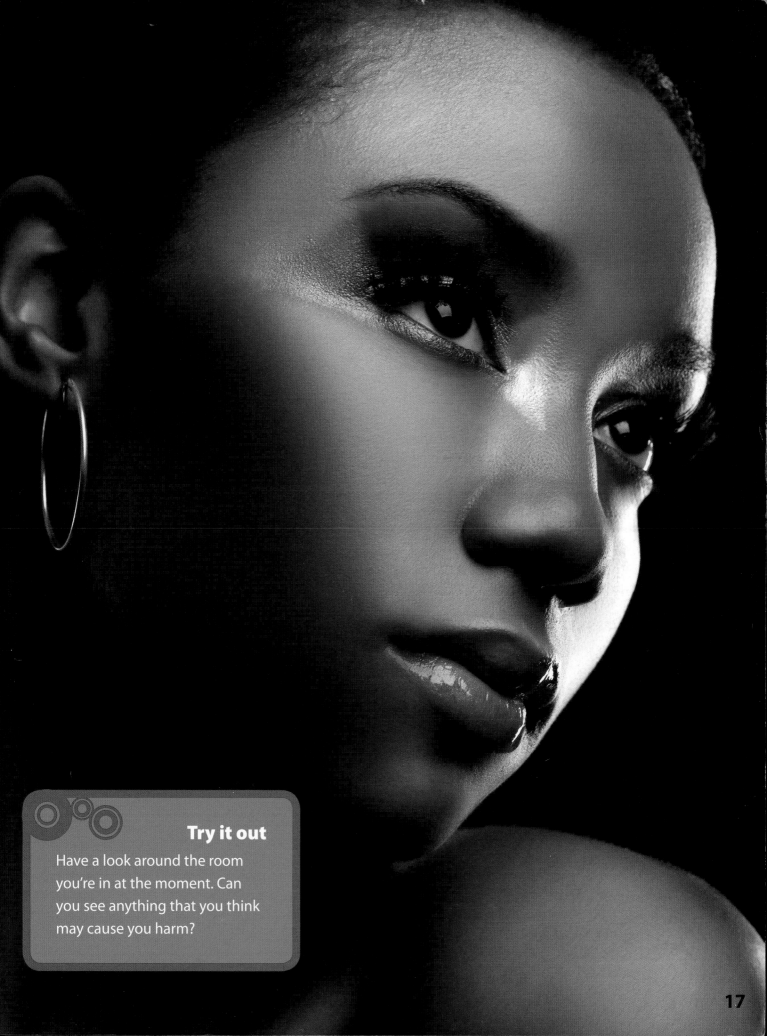

Try it out

Have a look around the room you're in at the moment. Can you see anything that you think may cause you harm?

Hazards and risks and the Health and Safety at Work Act

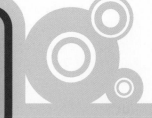

In this topic you will learn about:
- Hazards and risks in the workplace
- The Health and Safety at Work Act

Why do you think that hair and beauty salons have to be kept clean and tidy? What might happen if a salon was allowed to get untidy and dirty?

Hazards and risks

You will find the words hazards and risks discussed frequently. It's important you know what they mean and the difference between them.

- A hazard is something that could possibly cause an accident or an injury. For example, water on the floor is a hazard as it could cause someone to slip and fall.
- A risk is the likelihood (how likely something is to happen) that an accident might occur. For example, how likely is it that someone might slip on the water that has been spilled on the floor?

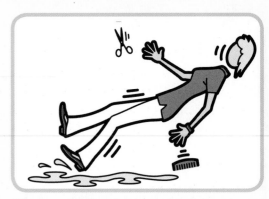

Water on the floor is a hazard and there is a risk that someone may slip and fall.

Health and Safety at Work Act

This is the main health and safety law. All employers have to make sure the salon is a safe place for you to work. There are lots of different ways they can do this.

Employers' responsibilities

- To provide a safe place to work
- To provide good entrances and exits for the salon
- To keep humidity levels acceptable
- To provide safe tools and equipment to use
- To provide safe methods of storing, handling and recognising hazardous substances like chemicals
- To provide protective clothing
- To provide information, instruction, training and supervision of employees – the workers
- To make sure the salon is the right temperature to work in
- To report accidents in the right way
- To make sure there are clean toilets and wash areas
- To make sure there are good evacuation plans in place, including an assembly point
- To make sure the salon is properly ventilated so the air is fresh and well circulated to prevent problems with fumes and dust
- To keep a fully stocked first aid box

The salon has to have its own health and safety policy. This sets out the rules the employer must follow to make sure all employees and clients are safe. Your employer must review the policy at regular intervals to make sure it's working well.

There will also be rules that *you* have to follow. You must make sure that no one gets harmed because of things you do, or don't do. If you notice a hazard, try to deal with it immediately. If you can't, report it to your employer. For example, if you notice there is hair on the floor, sweep it up straight away. If you don't, someone might slip and fall and hurt themselves.

Most accidents in the salon are caused by slips, trips and falls.

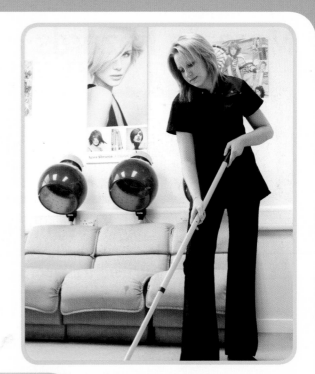

In the salon

Ami was a fun-loving junior in a busy salon. She loved salon life and enjoyed chatting to the clients. The only down side was her manager – Ami always seemed to be in trouble. He was always reminding her about health and safety but she couldn't understand why it was so important.

Part of Ami's role was to keep the salon clean and tidy and put things away. One of the stylists had just finished with the straightening irons and asked Ami to them to turn them off and put them away – but she didn't. A client had brought her young son into the salon and, when no one was looking, he picked them up and burned his hand very badly.

- Was Ami at fault? Do you think the manager would be in trouble?

Try it out

Has your salon got a health and safety policy? Get a copy and write down any important information you find in it.

 Functional skills
English

Just checking

1 An example of a hazard could be:
   a A hairdryer
   b Tweezers
   c Hair on the floor
   d Tiles on the floor.

2 Most accidents in the salon are caused by:
   a Slips, trips and hops
   b Hop, skip and jumps
   c Slips, trips and falls
   d Trips, journeys and jumps.

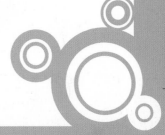

More on hazards and risks

Q If you spot a bottle of nail varnish remover with its top off, what should you do to make sure everyone in the salon is safe? Why do you think it's important?

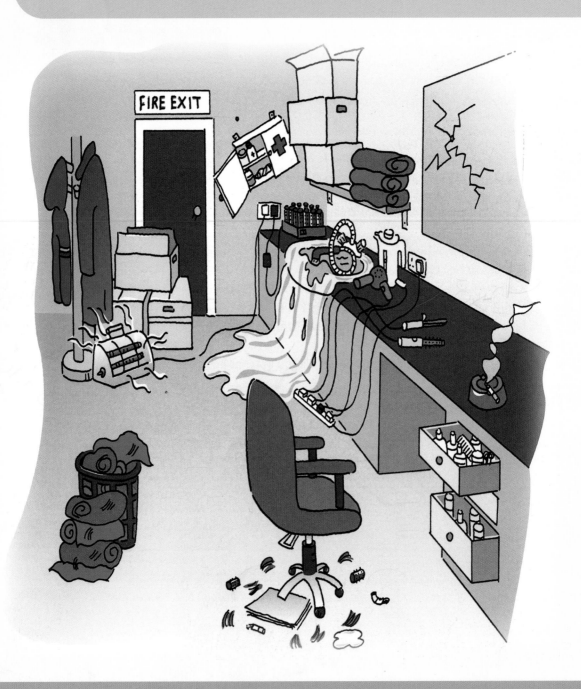

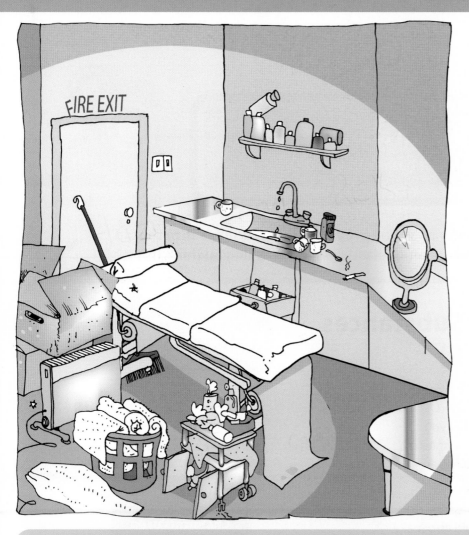

Try it out

Make a table (as below) and then:

1 write down the hazards you can see in both pictures.
2 decide what could happen if you didn't do anything about it.
3 suggest what you think you should do about it.

An example has been given to help you.

Hazard	What might happen?	What should I do?
Water on the floor	Someone might slip and fall	Mop it up straight away

 Functional skills – English writing

Just checking

1 Sweeping up hair cuttings from the floor will help to stop accidents from happening. True or false?
2 A wax pot that is left on and unattended is safe. True or false?

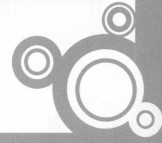

COSHH

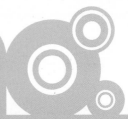

Q When you buy hair colouring products from the shops they should always come with a pair of plastic gloves. Why do you think this is?

COSHH (Control Of Substances Hazardous to Health)

When we talk about COSHH, we mean chemicals. All chemicals should be stored, handled, used and disposed of correctly. It is essential that you follow the manufacturer's instructions. Examples of the kinds of chemicals that are used in salons are shown here (right).

Your employer has a responsibility to assess the risk to your health and safety. He or she should also make sure you know how to store, handle, use and dispose of these chemicals in a safe way.

Eyelash and eyebrow tint: tint used for colouring the lashes or brows

Hair colourant: used in salons for dying hair

Perm lotion: lotion used to make straight hair curly

Chemicals used in salons

Nail polish remover

Relaxers: products used for straightening curly hair

Hydrogen peroxide: a chemical which helps colours and bleach to work

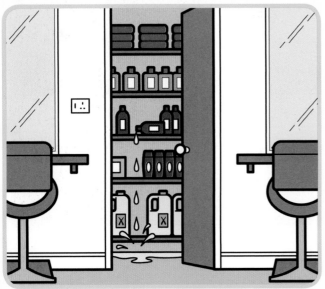

Poisonous or flammable chemicals are hazards and may present a high risk. However, if they are kept in a properly designed secure store, and handled by professionally trained people, the risk is much less.

Top tip

Chemicals and other products in the salon may be harmful. If you're not sure how to use them properly, ask your employer.

Product manufacturers should provide salons with information about how to work safely with chemicals and products. They will let your employer know the possible risks when using the products and what to do about them.

10A Hair Colorant – Semi-Permanent (Non-Aerosol)

Composition
Solutions of direct dyestuffs in a shampoo base which may be liquid, cream or gel.

Ingredients
Dyestuffs – up to 10%
Solvents (e.g. glycols or glycol ethers) – up to 10%
Ethanol – up to 50%

Hazards Identification
Refer to manufacturer's pack list of declarable dyestuffs which, if present, may require a sensitivity test before use. May be flammable.

First aid measures
Eyes: Rinse eyes immediately with plenty of water. If irritation persists, seek medical advice.
Skin: Wash skin immediately (mainly to avoid staining).
Ingestion: Drink 2–3 glasses of water or milk. Seek medical advice immediately.

Accidental release measures
Use plenty of water to dilute and mop up spillages.

Fire-fighting measures
Use carbon-dioxide or dry powder extinguisher.

Handling and storage
Avoid contact with eyes and face. Do not use on abraded or sensitive skin. Store in a cool place away from direct sunlight and other sources of heat. Use away from sources of ignition.
Liquid products may contain alcohol which makes the product flammable; keep small quantities in the salon for immediate use only.

Exposure Controls/ Personal Protection
Apply in a well-ventilated area. Always wear suitable protective gloves.

Disposal
Do not incinerate. Wash down the drain with plenty of water.

Nail polish remover

Composition
Liquid.

Ingredients
Ethyl acetate
Isopropyl alcohol
Water

Hazards Identification
Refer to manufacturer's instructions. May be flammable. Known irritant. Avoid inhalation.

First Aid Measures
Eyes: Flush out immediately with plenty of cold water. If irritation persists, seek medical advice.
Skin: Rinse immediately with cold water. If irritation persists, seek medical advice.

Accidental Release Measures
Absorb with tissue. Seal in a plastic bag for commercial waste disposal.

Fire-fighting Measures
Dry powder extinguisher.

Handling & Storage
Avoid contact with eyes and face. Do not use on abraded or sensitive skin. Store in a cool place away from direct sunlight and other sources of heat. Use away from sources of ignition.

Exposure Controls/ Personal Protection
Apply in a well ventilated area.

Disposal
Wash down the drain with plenty of cold water.

Examples of hazard data sheets giving information about chemical substances used in hair and beauty salons

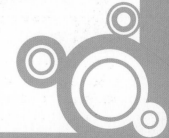

Try it out
Make a list of household items you can find with COSHH symbols.

Functional skills
English

Just checking
1 Where should poisonous or flammable chemicals be kept when they are not being used?
2 State four examples of products used in a hair and beauty salon that should be used following COSHH Regulations.

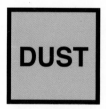
Dust

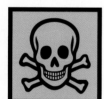
Toxic

Flammable

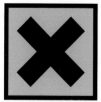
Irritant

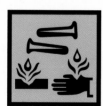
Corrosive

Oxidising agent

COSHH symbols

A lot of household products are also hazardous. Those that are hazardous will have COSHH symbols on them.

PPE and the Electricity at Work Regulations

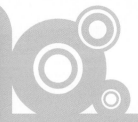

Q What kind of electrical equipment would you use in a hairdressing or beauty salon?

PPE (Personal Protective Equipment)

Most of the chemicals you come into contact with in the salon can be harmful if they're not used properly. Part of your employer's job is to make sure you know how to work safely with chemicals and other products that may be hazardous.

When you are working with hazardous substances, you should be wearing personal protective equipment (PPE). This would usually be:

- gloves to protect your hands
- an apron to protect your clothes.

You may also need to wear an apron and gloves if you're helping with a waxing service in the beauty salon. This is because sometimes the client's skin may bleed a little. The apron will protect your uniform and the gloves will protect any cuts on your hands.

Top tip

Your gloves are very important. They can help to stop you developing **dermatitis** and prevent cross-infection.

Key terms

Epilation – removing hair from the body by using a needle and an electrical current

Dermatitis – inflammation of the skin

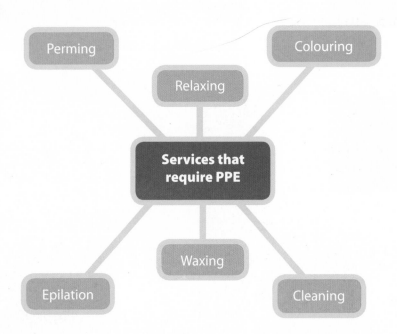

Perming

Colouring

Relaxing

Services that require PPE

Waxing

Epilation

Cleaning

Electricity at Work Regulations

Your employer has to make sure you have safe equipment to use in the salon. All electrical equipment should be tested at least once a year by a qualified electrician.

Before you use any electrical equipment you need to check that it is safe. To do this, check that:

- the **flex** isn't frayed or split
- plugs and sockets aren't broken or cracked
- hairdryers have an air filter attached to them
- you know how to use the equipment safely.

Remember – if you don't know how to use the equipment, ask!

Electrical hazards

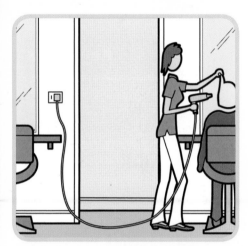

A trailing electrical cable is a hazard. If it is lying across a walkway there is a high risk of someone tripping over it. However, if it lies flat to the floor alongside the wall, the risk is much less.

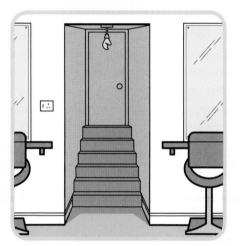

A failed light bulb is a hazard. If it is just one bulb out of many in a room, it presents very little risk, but if it is the only light on a staircase, it is a very high risk.

Key term

Flex – the wire that goes from the equipment to the plug

Top tips

If you have used electrical equipment, for example, straightening irons or a wax pot, make sure it has cooled down before you put it away.

If you find any electrical equipment is faulty when you're checking it you should:

- put a 'faulty' label or sticker on the equipment immediately
- take the equipment out of the salon and store it safely
- report it to the manager or salon owner.

Just checking

1 You should be wearing your PPE when you are:
   a Drying hair
   b Painting nails
   c Cleaning the salon
   d Combing hair.

2 If you are following Electricity at Work Regulations, you should:
   a Use all electrical equipment
   b Report, label and remove any faulty equipment
   c Wash all electrical equipment before you use it
   d Follow COSHH Regulations.

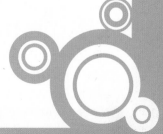

Good posture and safe handling

In this topic you will learn about:
- Good posture
- Safe handling techniques

 How could sitting in a slouched position for long periods of time affect your back as you get older?

Posture is about the way you sit or stand. Your posture in the salon is very important. If your posture isn't good, you may find your neck and shoulders ache and are stiff by the evening. It will also make you feel tired more quickly. You may not notice any of these problems now when you are young and your body is quite **flexible**, but when you get older, you could end up with **severe** back pain.

When you are standing, you should stand up straight with your feet slightly apart and your weight evenly distributed (for example, don't stand with all your weight on one leg). If you're sitting down, you should sit up straight with your back against the back of the chair and your feet on the floor or on a foot rest.

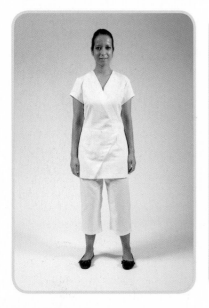
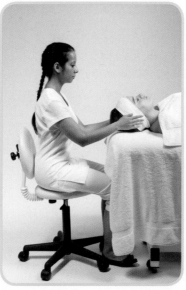

Good standing and sitting posture

Lifting objects safely

This comes under the **legislation** Manual Handling Operations Regulations. Your employer should make sure you are trained to lift heavy objects safely. An example may be a box of stock that has just been delivered and needs to be moved somewhere.

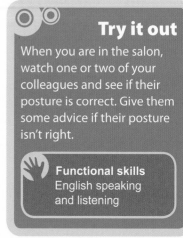

Key terms

Flexible – able to bend easily
Severe – very bad

Try it out

When you are in the salon, watch one or two of your colleagues and see if their posture is correct. Give them some advice if their posture isn't right.

Functional skills
English speaking and listening

Key term

Legislation – law

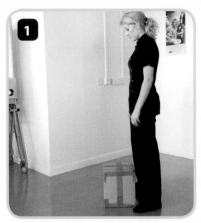

Think about the lift. Where is the load to be placed? Do you need help? Are handling aids available?

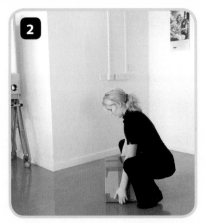

With your feet close to the load, bend your knees and keep your back straight. Tuck in your chin. Lean forward slightly over the load to get a good grip.

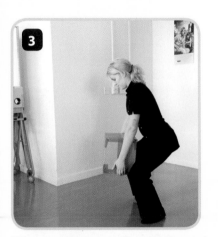

When you are sure of your grip on the load, straighten your legs and lift smoothly. Remember to keep your back straight.

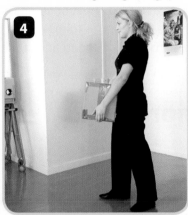

Carry the load close to your body.

Top tip

If you think the object that needs to be moved is too heavy, ask someone to help you.

Key terms

Sturdy – strong
Colleagues – workmates

If you need to lift a large or heavy object from a shelf, make sure you use a **sturdy** stepladder. Hold the object firmly, keeping it close to your body before you climb down the steps. You could ask one of your **colleagues** to hold the stepladder to make sure it doesn't move.

Just checking

1 How can you recognise that someone has good posture?
    a Slouching
    b Standing on one leg
    c Standing up straight with their feet slightly apart
    d Standing with bent knees

2 How should you lift a heavy object?
    a Bend your knees and get a good grip of the object. Stand up, keeping the object close to your body.
    b Bend forward; get a good grip of the object and stand up.
    c Bend your knees, lean forward and grip the object with one hand and use the other hand to pull yourself up.
    d Bend down, curling your back, grip the box and stand up using the muscles in your back.

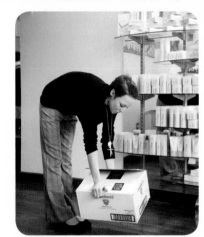

A heavy box is a hazard. It can present a high risk to someone who lifts it incorrectly (as shown), rather than someone who uses the correct manual handling techniques.

Sterilising equipment

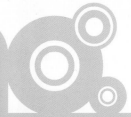

Why do think it is important that all tools and equipment that will be used in a hairdressing or beauty salon are clean for every client?

Sterilisation is the destruction of all germs and bacteria by heat or chemicals. It is important that all tools used in the salon are free from germs to make sure that everyone is safe. Therefore it is essential that all tools are cleaned and sterilised before use. This is to stop **cross-infection**.

Methods of sterilisation and disinfection

The autoclave

Steam sterilising (using an autoclave) is the most effective method of sterilisation. It is used for metal tools such as scissors, tweezers, etc.

The chemical jar (barbicide)

The chemical jar is used widely in both hairdressing and beauty salons. You should read and follow the manufacturer's instructions when making up the solution. Remember it should be changed every day. All tools should be fully **immersed** in the solution and left for the time specified by the manufacturer. The chemical jar will only work to disinfect your tools – it won't kill all the germs.

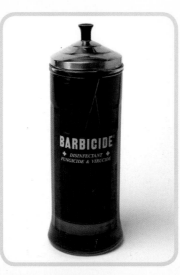

> **Key term**
>
> **Cross-infection** – passing germs from one person to another

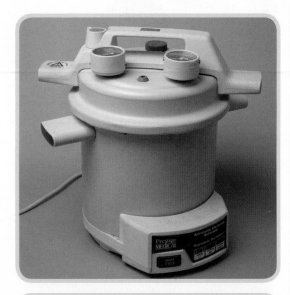

> **Top tip**
>
> An autoclave works like a pressure cooker and reaches a very high temperature. You must make sure it has cooled down before you remove your tools or you may burn or scald yourself.

> **Key term**
>
> **Immersed** – covered by the solution

The UV (ultra-violet) cabinet

The UV cabinet is another method that you may use in the salon. The ultra-violet rays (like those on a sun bed) can be used to disinfect tools. Your tools should be clean and dry when placed in the UV cabinet. Turn them every 20 minutes to stop the growth of bacteria.

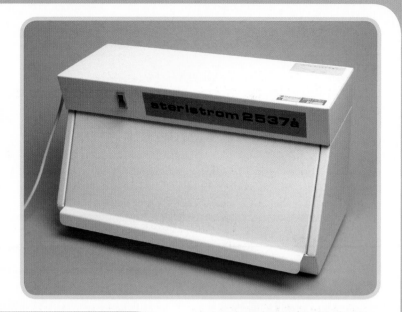

In the salon

Saima had been working in the beauty salon for 6 weeks. She enjoyed helping the therapists set up for the treatments and looking after the clients.

She didn't really like all the cleaning that she had to do, but she understood that the salon and its equipment had to be really clean and hygienic. She seemed to spend quite a lot of her working day cleaning and sterilising tools ready for the therapists. She also had to make sure the salon was spotless.

One day she noticed her hands were really itchy and quite sore. The following day it was just as bad. It got even worse when she started cleaning the salon. A week later they were so sore that she thought she ought to tell the manager – each time she started to clean she wanted to cry because her hands hurt so much.

- What do you think was wrong with Saima's hands? What should she have done to stop this from happening?

Try it out

Ask your tutor to show you how to use each of the sterilisers. When you feel confident, sterilise a comb and some tweezers. Ask your tutor to watch you and give you feedback on how well you did.

Just checking

1 What is the most effective method of sterilisation?
  a The autoclave
  b The chemical jar
  c Soapy detergents
  d The UV cabinet

2 Sterilisation is:
  a The destruction of all germs and bacteria
  b The destruction of all macro organisms
  c The growth of micro organisms
  d The deterioration of macro organisms.

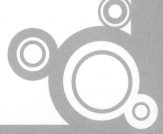

Emotions and first aid

In this topic you will learn about:

- Evacuation during an emergency
- First aid

 Q Why is it important that you know what to do if there is an emergency when you are working in a salon?

Evacuation

There may be times when you have to **evacuate** the salon quickly (for example, if there is a fire or a bomb alert). It is important that you know what to do and where to go to make sure that you are safe and also to make sure that everyone else is safe too.

When you evacuate the salon you should leave quickly without running. Don't stop to get your personal possessions, for example, your coat, mobile phone, etc. If you do, it will take you longer to get out of the salon.

You should follow the fire exit signs and go to the assembly point outside the building (you should know where this is).

The assembly point is where everyone who has evacuated the building should meet. This is to make sure that everyone is accounted for. If anyone is missing, the fire service will be told when they arrive and they will go in and rescue anyone left in the building.

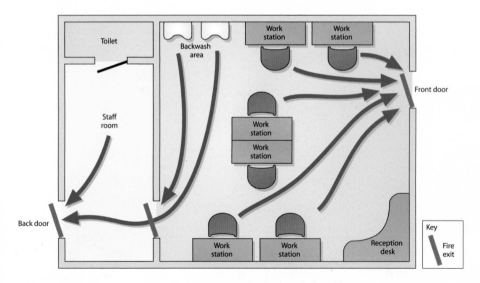

An evacuation plan for a hairdressing salon

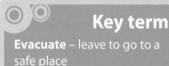

Key term

Evacuate – leave to go to a safe place

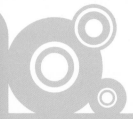

Top tip

When you are evacuating the clients from a salon, the appointment book should be taken to the assembly point. This is so that someone can check that all the clients are safe.

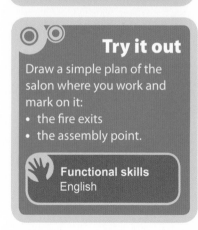

Try it out

Draw a simple plan of the salon where you work and mark on it:

- the fire exits
- the assembly point.

Functional skills
English

First aid

All salons must have a first aid box. Someone must be responsible for making sure it has the right items in it and that it is kept fully stocked. You should know where the first aid kit is kept in your salon.

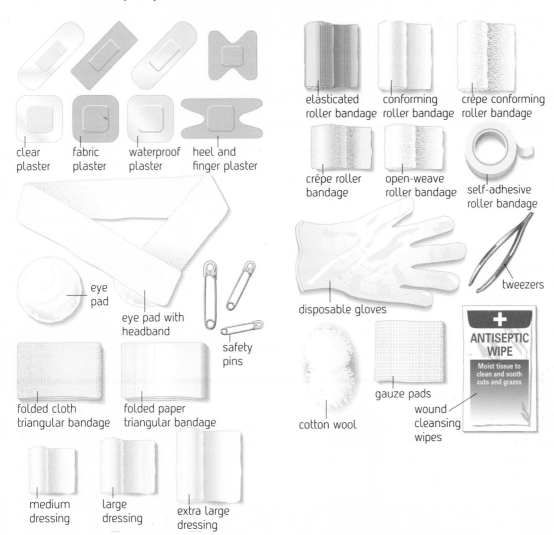

clear plaster

fabric plaster

waterproof plaster

heel and finger plaster

elasticated roller bandage

conforming roller bandage

crêpe conforming roller bandage

crêpe roller bandage

open-weave roller bandage

self-adhesive roller bandage

eye pad

eye pad with headband

safety pins

disposable gloves

tweezers

folded cloth triangular bandage

folded paper triangular bandage

cotton wool

gauze pads

ANTISEPTIC WIPE
Moist tissue to clean and sooth cuts and grazes

wound cleansing wipes

medium dressing

large dressing

extra large dressing

Just checking

1 When evacuating the salon because there is a fire, should you stop to get your mobile phone?
   a Yes, because you might need to call your mum or dad.
   b Yes, because your friends will want to know all the gossip.
   c No, because you might end up getting trapped in the building.
   d Yes, it cost a lot of money.

2 Which of the following would be some of the correct items you would find in a first aid kit?
   a Bandages, plasters and a fork
   b Antiseptic wipes and drawing pins
   c Plasters, cotton wool and bandages
   d An eye patch, safety pins and a tint brush.

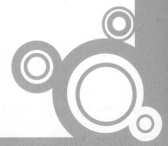

Fire safety and fire extinguishers

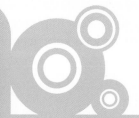

In this topic you will learn about:

- Fire safety
- The different types of fire extinguisher

Q Can you use any fire extinguisher on a fire?

Fire safety

You need to know where all the fire extinguishers are in the salon. There are different types of extinguishers that should be used on different types of fires. All fire extinguishers should be red with a different coloured area that tells you what it contains.

Top tip

If you use the wrong type of extinguisher on a fire, you could make the fire worse. You could even cause serious injuries to yourself or someone else.
The salon may also have a fire blanket. These can be used to smother flames. They are especially good for wrapping around someone who is on fire.

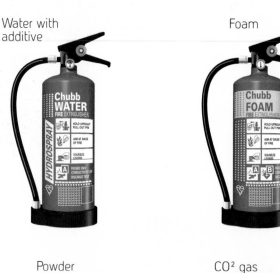

Water with additive

Foam

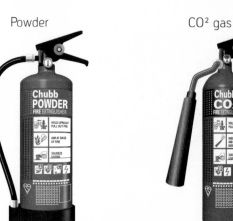

Powder

CO_2 gas

Types of fire extinguisher

Extinguisher	Colour	What it is used for	Do not use on
Water	RED	Wood, paper and fabric material	Liquid, electrical or metal fires
Powder	BLUE	Liquid and electrical fires	Metal fires
Foam	YELLOW	Liquid fires	Electrical or metal fires
Carbon dioxide	BLACK	Liquid and electrical fires	Metal fires

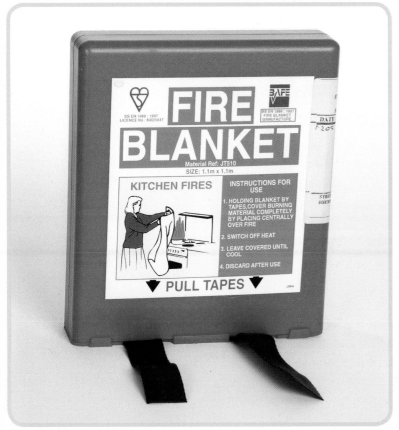

A fire blanket

Try it out

Use the simple plan of the salon's fire exits and the fire assembly point that you made earlier (see page 30). Mark where you will find:

- fire extinguishers, using the colour codes of each extinguisher (for example, if you have a water extinguisher, mark it in red)
- the fire blanket (if the salon has one)
- the first aid kit.

Functional skills
English reading and writing

Just checking

1 If there is a paper fire, the correct extinguisher to use would be:
   a Red
   b Blue
   c Yellow
   d Black.

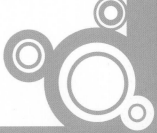

Presenting a professional image in a salon

In this unit you will learn about:

- How to present a professional image
- How to maintain personal hygiene
- Good communication in the salon
- How to act professionally in the salon

Introduction

Your **professional image** is very important when you are working in a salon **environment**. Clients will make judgements about the salon by the way you look and act. So you should always be dressed and presented professionally so that clients want to come into your salon.

Top tip

Always be well presented. Your image is important to the salon. If clients don't think you look the part, they may go elsewhere. This means the salon could lose money, and you could lose your job!

Key terms

Professional image – looking clean, tidy and presentable (both you and the salon)

Environment – what is around you (your surroundings)

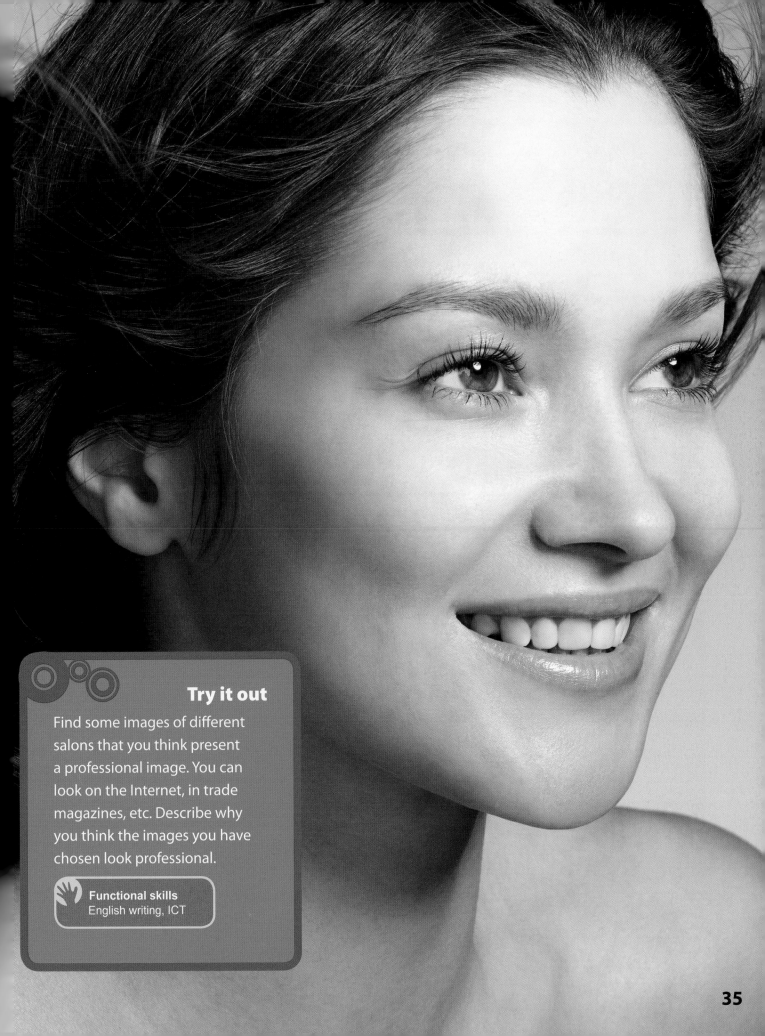

Try it out

Find some images of different salons that you think present a professional image. You can look on the Internet, in trade magazines, etc. Describe why you think the images you have chosen look professional.

Functional skills
English writing, ICT

35

Present a professional image

In this topic you will learn about:

- How to promote and present a professional image in a salon

Q Find an image of a salon environment that would make you feel at ease as a client. Use magazines or the Internet. Describe what you like about it and how you think the staff should look.

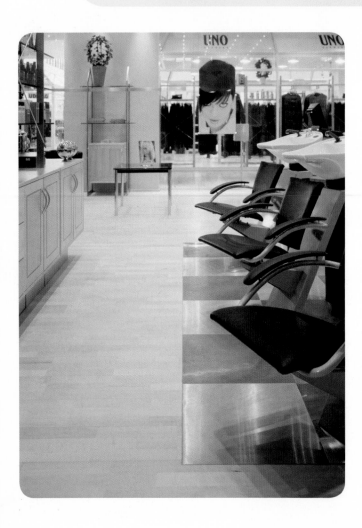

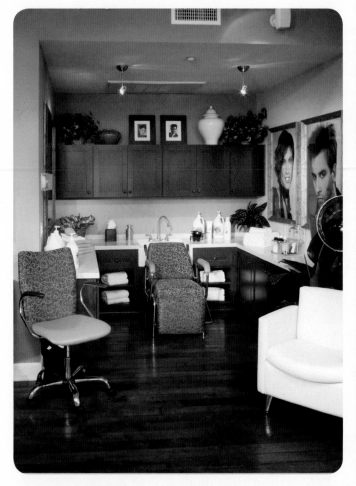

Try it out

What is it about these two salons that looks so professional? Are they clean, tidy and modern? What is it exactly that you like? Would you be happy to work in one of them and if so why?

There are many different types of salon around. They range from very trendy ones to more traditional salons, with all the others in between. The image of a salon is aimed at the type of clients it is trying to attract. For example, a trendy salon will want to attract younger clients than one where most of the clients are elderly.

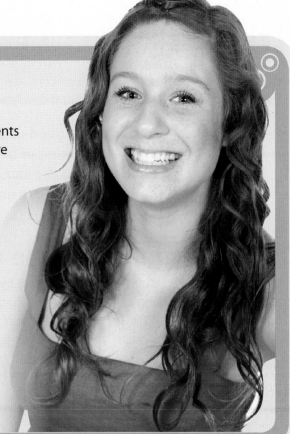

In the salon

Keeley had been working in the salon for a few weeks. The manager told her that she had received complaints from clients about the way she dressed. She told her that her T-shirts were too skimpy and that her heels were too high. Clients felt embarrassed when she was shampooing because she was showing too much skin. Plus there was a risk of injury because of her heels. Keeley loved the way she dressed but loved her job more. She decided to cover up when she was in the salon and wear lower heeled shoes.

- Do you think Keeley was right to change the way she dressed? Why?

Just checking

1 What do you think the term 'professional image' means?
2 How can you make sure you present a professional image at all times?
   a Keep the salon clean and tidy.
   b Sit down at every opportunity you get to have a rest.
   c Check your hair and make-up regularly and smarten as needed.
   d Leave the cleaning for someone less busy than you are.

Top tip

If you have a spare moment in the salon, take a look at yourself in the mirror and adjust your hair or make-up to look presentable. Check out the salon surroundings and clean or tidy up anything you notice is dirty or out of place. This is called 'using your initiative' and your employer will be very impressed.

How to maintain personal hygiene

Q

Do you have a good daily personal hygiene routine? Does it involve showering or bathing every day? This is a standard requirement in the hair and beauty industry. It's essential to present a fresh, clean image!

Daily personal hygiene routine

It is important that you look after your **personal hygiene** when working in a salon. You will be working quite close to your clients so if you have body odour or bad breath it will be very unpleasant for them. To make sure you smell fresh every day you must have a daily cleansing routine.

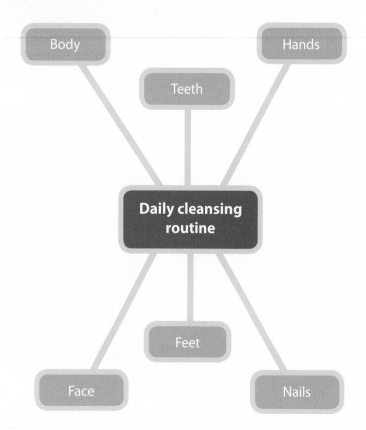

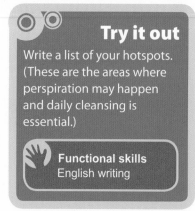

Key term

Personal hygiene – cleaning your body parts that may perspire (sweat) or smell unpleasant

Try it out

Write a list of your hotspots. (These are the areas where perspiration may happen and daily cleansing is essential.)

Functional skills
English writing

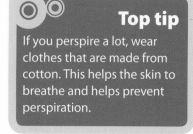

Top tip

If you perspire a lot, wear clothes that are made from cotton. This helps the skin to breathe and helps prevent perspiration.

The table below offers some advice on how to maintain personal freshness.

Potential hotspot	How to maintain freshness
Underarms and pubic region	Shower or bathe everyday and use an antiperspirant under the arms or a feminine hygiene spray or powder around the pubic region.
Feet	Shower or bathe every day and wear cotton socks and leather shoes if your feet perspire.
Teeth	Brush your teeth twice a day (or even more) and use a freshener spray or mouthwash to freshen your breath.
Hands	Wash them regularly, especially after using the toilet. Use a hygiene hand rub regularly.
Nails	Regular washing of hands should ensure clean nails. Wear gloves if you are using colour to avoid staining the nail.
Face	Cleanse, tone and moisturise every day and thoroughly remove make-up to help prevent spots and greasy skin.

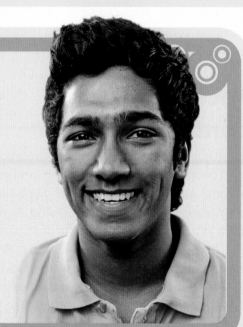

In the salon

Navin had been at his new salon for just a week when he was confronted by the salon manager. Apparently a few clients had complained that Navin smelt of cigarettes when he was shampooing their hair. The manager said he would either have to stop smoking while at work or make sure he freshened up fully after having a cigarette. Navin apologised and said he would stop smoking at work and chew nicotine gum instead. He said he was thinking of giving up anyway because of the cost.

- Why might a client complain about the smell of nicotine on their stylists or therapists? Do you think it is professional to smoke and then continue working in the salon and why? Do you notice or dislike the smell of smoke on other people?

Just checking

1 Which of the following are hotspots to be kept clean and fresh at all times?
   a Face
   b Legs
   c Underarms
   d Teeth

2 Who is responsible for your personal hygiene?

3 How can you make sure your breath always smells fresh?

Top tip

Keep a breath freshener spray at work and avoid eating anything that may have a strong smell, for example, onions, garlic or spicy foods.

Good communication in the salon

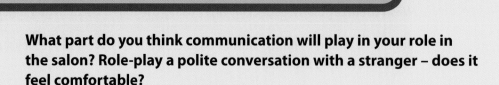

In this topic you will learn about:

- How to communicate clearly and professionally when working in a salon

Q What part do you think communication will play in your role in the salon? Role-play a polite conversation with a stranger – does it feel comfortable?

Communication skills can be broken down into two main types:

- Verbal communication – talking to clients either face to face or on the telephone
- Non-verbal communication – body language, hand gestures and facial expression.

Face-to-face communication

There is a lot of face-to-face communication in the salon, both between staff and with clients, and you need to become good at it. Eye contact shows a client that you are interested in what they are saying. If you cannot give them your full attention because of something else, excuse yourself politely and deal with it. But you must remember to return and not get sidetracked! Speak clearly – don't put your hands in front of your face or chew gum or sweets. If you are struggling to understand what a client wants, ask a senior member of staff for help – this is being professional.

Body language can be both **open** and **closed**. If it is open you will look relaxed with your arms and legs uncrossed. However, if your body language is closed, you may look angry and unwelcoming. For example, sitting with your arms folded or your head in your hands gives a very negative impression of your mood. Your posture is important too – slouching across the reception desk because you are tired looks very unprofessional.

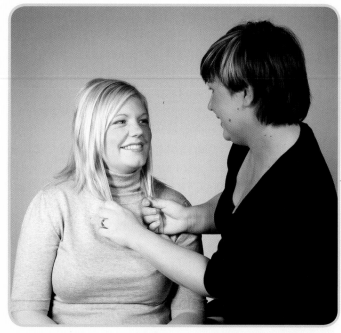

By being at the client's eye level and smiling, you give a friendly impression and put the client at their ease

Key terms

Open body language – showing by your posture and gestures that you are relaxed and welcoming
Closed body language – the opposite of open body language, where your posture and gestures show that you are tense and negative

Telephone communication

Find out the correct greeting for your salon. It will probably be something like this,

'Good morning/afternoon, Hair Academy, Natalie speaking, how can I help you?'

It is important to smile when you speak on the telephone because it gives a friendly **tone** to your voice. It will also show clients and salon staff that you are being polite in your telephone manner. Never hang up on a caller. If you don't feel you can deal with the enquiry, ask them to hold the line while you pass it over to a senior member of staff.

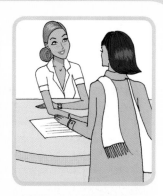

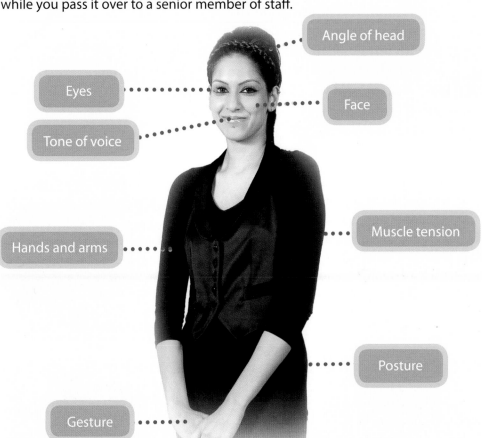

- Angle of head
- Eyes
- Face
- Tone of voice
- Muscle tension
- Hands and arms
- Posture
- Gesture

Non-verbal communication is expressed through your body language and facial expressions

Try it out

Look at these two illustrations above. Which one shows an open body language and which one shows a closed body language? Why? How would you feel when greeted in the salon by each of these?

Key term

Tone of voice – the way your voice sounds; for example, quiet, loud, angry, happy

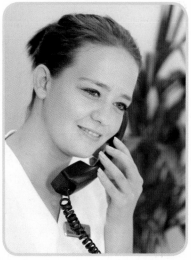

Smile when you speak on the phone – the client will be able to hear it in your voice

Just checking

1 Why is it important to look at a client when they are talking to you?
   - a So they think you are interested in what they are saying
   - b To stop you being bored
   - c To help you understand what they are saying
   - d So you can check if they need a haircut or facial

2 Why is the way you talk both face to face and over the telephone important for the salon's professional image?

Acting professionally in the salon

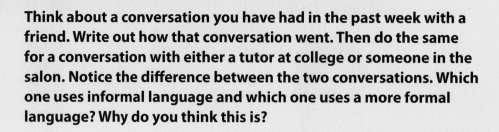

In this topic you will learn about:

- How to act professionally when working in a salon

Q Think about a conversation you have had in the past week with a friend. Write out how that conversation went. Then do the same for a conversation with either a tutor at college or someone in the salon. Notice the difference between the two conversations. Which one uses informal language and which one uses a more formal language? Why do you think this is?

In the salon, you must always take care with your facial expressions and body language. Remember that you are surrounded by mirrors and anyone could be watching! You will only get one chance to make a positive impression and it is very important to both the salon and your own career that it is a good one. Never shout out in the salon, especially if you are asking a question for a client. Would you want everyone to know if you had just asked a personal question about a treatment such as bikini waxing? This is known as being tactful and discreet.

Key terms

Tactful – understanding what it is right to say or do without offending anyone

Discreet – being quiet about something that might cause someone embarrassment

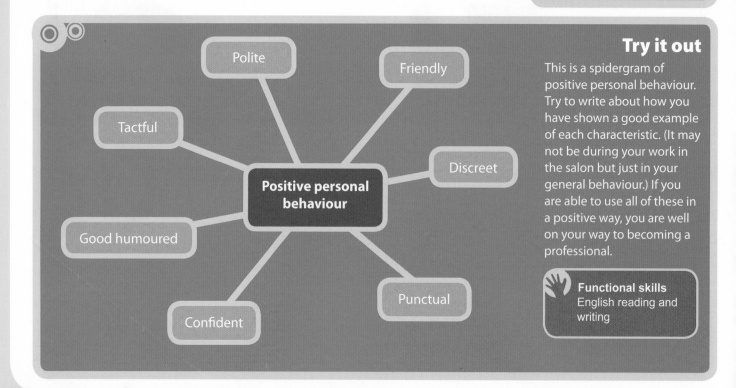

Try it out

This is a spidergram of positive personal behaviour. Try to write about how you have shown a good example of each characteristic. (It may not be during your work in the salon but just in your general behaviour.) If you are able to use all of these in a positive way, you are well on your way to becoming a professional.

Functional skills
English reading and writing

In the salon

A client came into the salon to complain that her fake tan was streaky. Shabeena told the client that it looked fine to her. The client became angry and told her to get the manager immediately. Shabeena thought the client was in the wrong and told her she would get the boss to come over and sort her out! However, her boss told Shabeena that she was in the wrong and made her apologise to the client.

- Who should apologise – the client to Shabeena or Shabeena to the client – and why? Would you have dealt with it yourself or brought a senior member of staff over straight away?

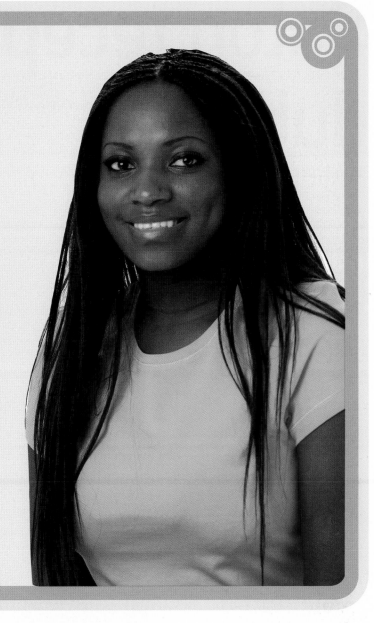

Just checking

1. Which of the following are good examples of positive personal behaviour?
   a Tactfulness
   b Tiredness
   c Shyness
   d Discretion

2. You are on the telephone when a client enters the salon. What should you do?
   a Ignore them and deal with the telephone enquiry first.
   b Acknowledge them, smile and carry on with the phone call.
   c Tell the caller on the phone to wait while you deal with the client.
   d Shout for someone else to deal with the person while you finish the call.

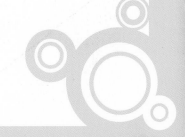

Salon reception duties

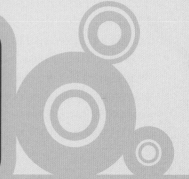

In this unit you will learn about:

- Carrying out salon reception duties
- The payment methods used for salon services
- Recording salon appointments

Introduction

Clients are likely to have their first experience of a salon in the reception area. Here they will first decide whether or not they are happy with the salon. So it is essential that it is **welcoming**, tidy and **professional** at all times.

If you are in the reception area, you must provide an excellent customer service. You should always be aware of clients entering the salon and greet them in a polite and friendly way. Use good **verbal** and **non-verbal communication skills**, even when under pressure. This helps to create an overall professional image of the salon.

You will be responsible for making client appointments and must learn how to use the **appointment system** correctly. You will also need to know how to take payments. All this will ensure that the salon runs smoothly through the working day.

Top tip

When you are on reception, always answer the telephone with a smile on your face. If you are smiling it can be heard through your voice and the person you are speaking to will feel comfortable and happy.

Key terms

Welcoming – greet someone in a friendly way

Professional – expert at the work you do

Verbal communication skills – spoken word

Non-verbal communication skills – facial expressions, body language, etc.

Appointment system – the way appointments are recorded for clients visiting the salon

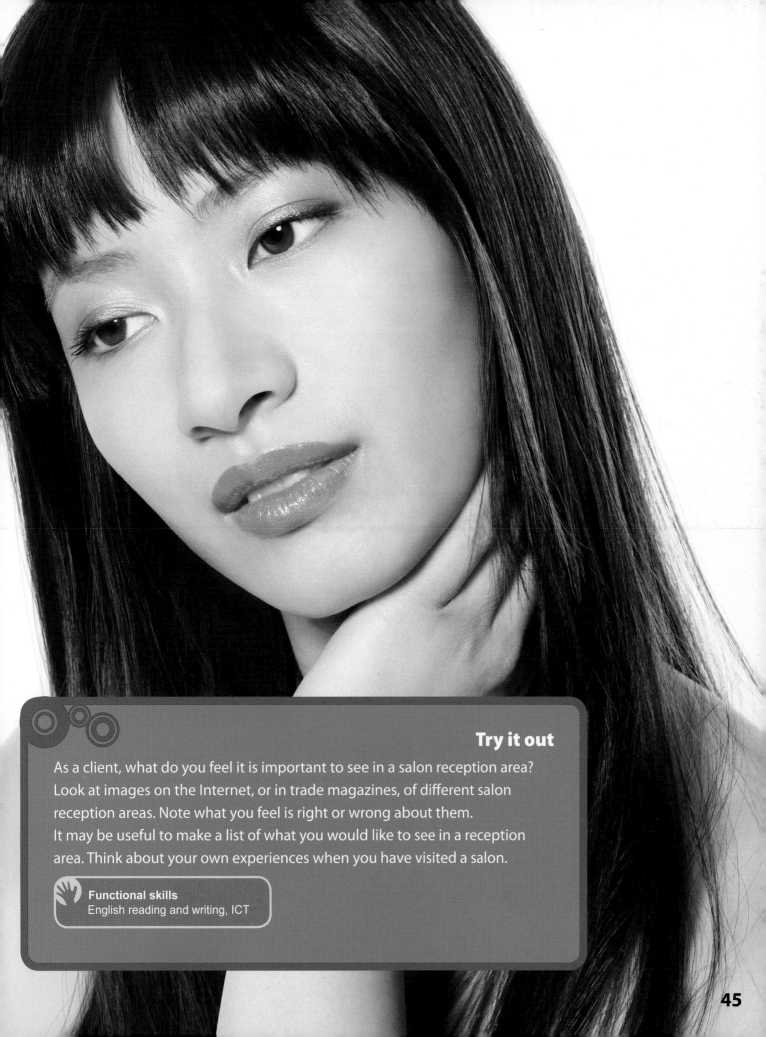

Try it out

As a client, what do you feel it is important to see in a salon reception area? Look at images on the Internet, or in trade magazines, of different salon reception areas. Note what you feel is right or wrong about them.

It may be useful to make a list of what you would like to see in a reception area. Think about your own experiences when you have visited a salon.

Functional skills
English reading and writing, ICT

Carrying out salon reception duties

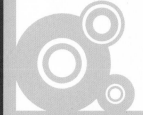

In this topic you will learn about:

- The need to present a positive image to the client
- Typical salon reception duties
- The **features** of a well-run reception service
- The importance of maintaining client confidentiality
- Payment methods used for salon services
- How to communicate and act within a salon environment

Q When you have been in a reception area for a salon, or any kind of business, what have you noticed the receptionist is doing as part of their job?

Check the unit *Presenting a professional image in a salon*. This gives you information on how to present a positive image to your clients. It also explains how to communicate and act professionally in a salon environment.

Reception duties

- Receiving clients
- Making appointments
- Checking appointments
- Promoting the sale of products, services and treatments
- **Reception duties**
- Offering services at reception – for example, beverages, magazines
- Taking care of clients' belongings
- Seating clients

Top tip

While you are on the reception area, remember to smile and be friendly. Offer to help – don't wait to be asked.

Key term

Features – the important parts

The features of a well-run reception service

While working on reception, you will need to tackle a variety of tasks. All of them will make the reception service run smoothly for both the client and the salon staff. At all times you should:

- deal with requests for appointments promptly
- record all messages correctly
- identify client requirements accurately
- check that the client is happy with the timing of their appointment
- make sure that information is passed on correctly to the right person.

Payment methods

Different salons accept different types of payment. The list below tells you all the methods that are available:

- cash
- cheque
- debit/credit card
- gift voucher.

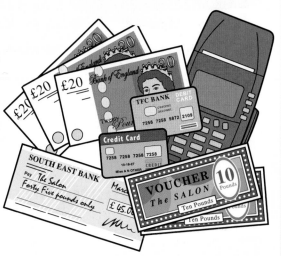

Maintaining client confidentiality

Client confidentiality means not discussing anything about a client with anyone other than the correct salon staff.

Top tip

If you have spare time while on reception, don't sit down – tidy up. A tidy reception area looks professional.

In the salon

Keeley was on her way to work on the bus and was discussing one of the salon's clients with her friend. She said that the client had terrible hair. However, a friend of the client was sitting nearby on the bus and overheard the conversation. She told the client who then complained to the salon. Keeley was given a formal, verbal warning for breach of client confidentiality and unprofessionalism.

- Why do you think the client complained about Keeley talking about her? How would you feel if you had been the client and someone was talking about you like this?

Try it out

List which payment methods are accepted in the salon where you work or are training. Are they different from any of the salons you have been in as a client?

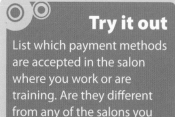

Functional skills
English writing

Just checking

1 Why do you need to smile and be helpful at reception?
   a To present a professional image of the salon
   b So that you feel good about yourself
   c So the client will give you a good tip
   d To make sure you keep the salon running on time

2 Which of the following are likely to be payment methods accepted in a salon?
   a Money b Cheque c An 'I owe you note' d Foreign currency

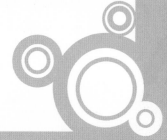

Recording salon appointments (1)

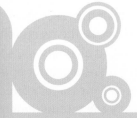

In this topic you will learn about:

- The basic information required from the client
- Recording appointments for a variety of services

 Think about the times when you have made an appointment in a salon – or when you have listened to someone else making an appointment. Make a list of the questions that the receptionist asked.

Basic information required from the client to make an appointment

When a client goes into a salon (or telephones) to make an appointment, there is some basic information that you must ask them.

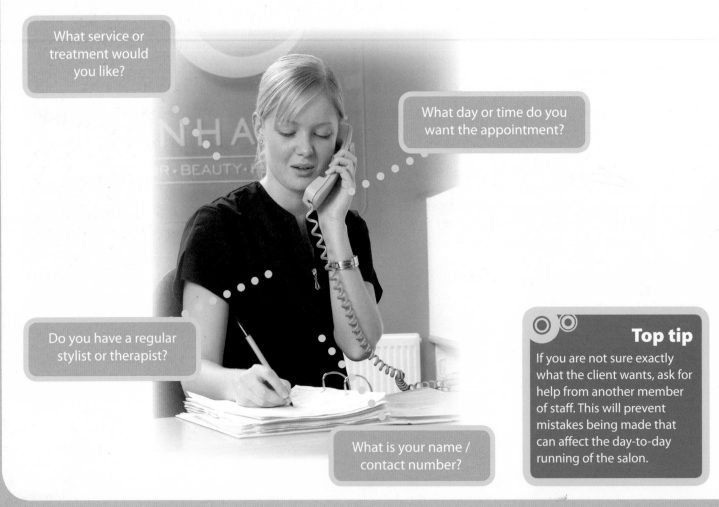

What service or treatment would you like?

What day or time do you want the appointment?

Do you have a regular stylist or therapist?

What is your name / contact number?

Top tip

If you are not sure exactly what the client wants, ask for help from another member of staff. This will prevent mistakes being made that can affect the day-to-day running of the salon.

Recording appointments for a variety of services

You will be observed by your assessor in the salon making appointments for clients. The checklist below will help you to remember exactly what the assessor is checking you can do correctly:

Observation point	How to carry it out correctly
Present a **positive image**	Be friendly, smile and follow the salon dress code.
Greet the client appropriately	Look at the client, smile and ask how you can help.
Record the salon appointment correctly	Take care to write in the appointment book correctly or enter the correct information into the computer.
Confirm the appointment with the client	Check back with the client and repeat all the details of the appointment you have made.
Communicate and behave in a professional manner	Be polite, smile, speak clearly, use good verbal and non-verbal communication skills.

Key terms

Positive image – the way you present yourself to the client

Greet – meeting a client initially, saying hello and welcoming them to the salon

Just checking

1 Which of the following questions might you ask when making an appointment for a client?
   a What treatment or service would you like?
   b What is your date of birth?
   c Do you have a contact telephone number?
   d Do you work close to the salon?

2 Which of the following are good examples of non-verbal communication?
   a Looking away while talking to your client
   b Listening to a member of staff talking while the client is speaking to you
   c Smiling and nodding to show you are listening
   d Yawning because you are bored

Try it out

Write out a list of the questions you need to ask when making an appointment for a client. Check these with your tutor/salon manager to see if you now know the salon procedure for making appointments.

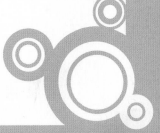

Functional skills
English writing

Recording salon appointments (2)

In this topic you will learn about:
- The different systems for recording appointments
- The factors to consider when agreeing appointment times

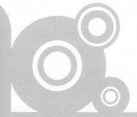

Q **What do you think the advantages and disadvantages of a written appointment book or a computerised appointment system might be?**

The different systems for recording appointments

The salon will either have an appointment book that you write in or use a computerised salon appointment system. Whichever it is, you will have to understand and use it correctly. It may take some time for you to learn how to do this and you should ask for help as you go along.

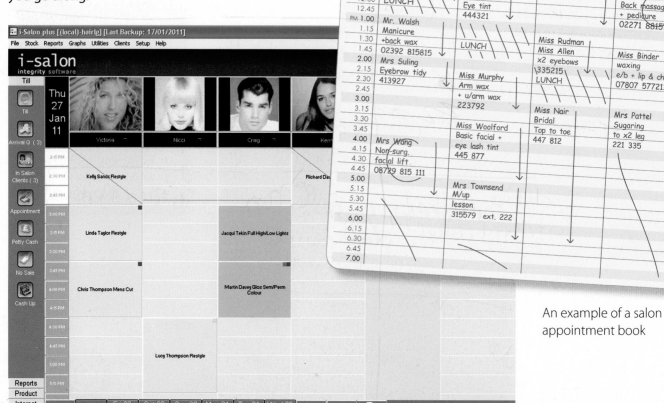

An example of a salon appointment book

An example of a page from a computerised appointment system

Factors to consider when agreeing appointment times

When you are agreeing appointment times with a client you should also consider:

- services and treatments available
- **typical duration**
- cost
- the need for appropriate **appointment spacing**.

In the salon

It was a busy afternoon in the beauty salon and Lian was rushing around trying to keep the salon tidy and running smoothly. A client came in – Lian remembered making a telephone appointment with her earlier that day. She greeted her and checked her appointment for a half leg wax. However, the client was expecting a full leg wax. The appointment was going to take longer than the time she had booked with the therapist. It meant the therapist would be running behind on a busy day.

- What do you think Lian had forgotten to do when she originally booked the appointment? How might the therapist feel, knowing that Lian had caused this disruption?

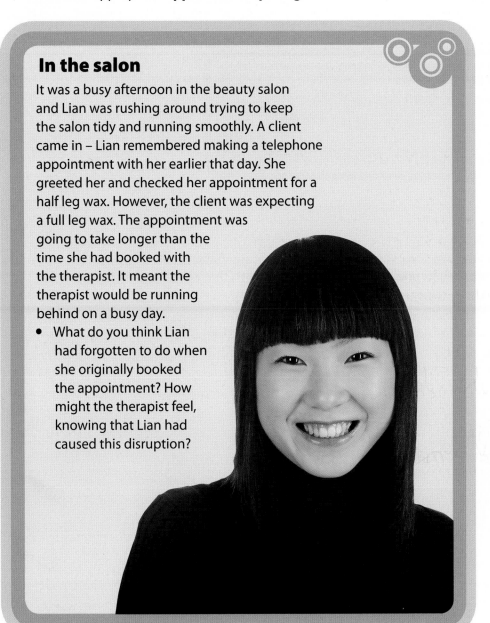

Key terms

Typical duration – the length of time a hairdressing service or beauty treatment may take

Appointment spacing – the time difference between the clients booked into the salon for their service or treatment

Try it out

Think about the list of factors to consider, above. Why is each of these important when you are agreeing the appointment time with your client? If you are unsure, ask another member of staff or your tutor.

Functional skills
English speaking and listening

Top tip

To ensure smooth running of the salon, take care with all entries made with appointments. If you are unsure always check with someone else.

Just checking

1. What are the two types of systems used to record salon appointments?
2. What does the term appropriate 'appointment spacing' mean?

Create an image using colour

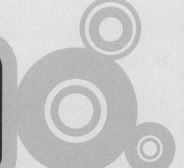

Introduction

This unit will help you to understand why the colour spectrum is important in the hair and beauty industry. You will learn about **primary** and **secondary colours**, and colours that cancel each other out. You will also discover how they can be used together to get the best look.

This will help you to choose the right make-up and hair colours to suit your skin tone. You will also be able to make sure the colour of your clothes works well with your hair and make-up.

Top tip

When you know and use the colours that suit your skin tones, you'll find your skin looks better and your eyes will sparkle!

Key terms

Primary colours – red, blue and yellow

Secondary colours – violet/purple, orange and green

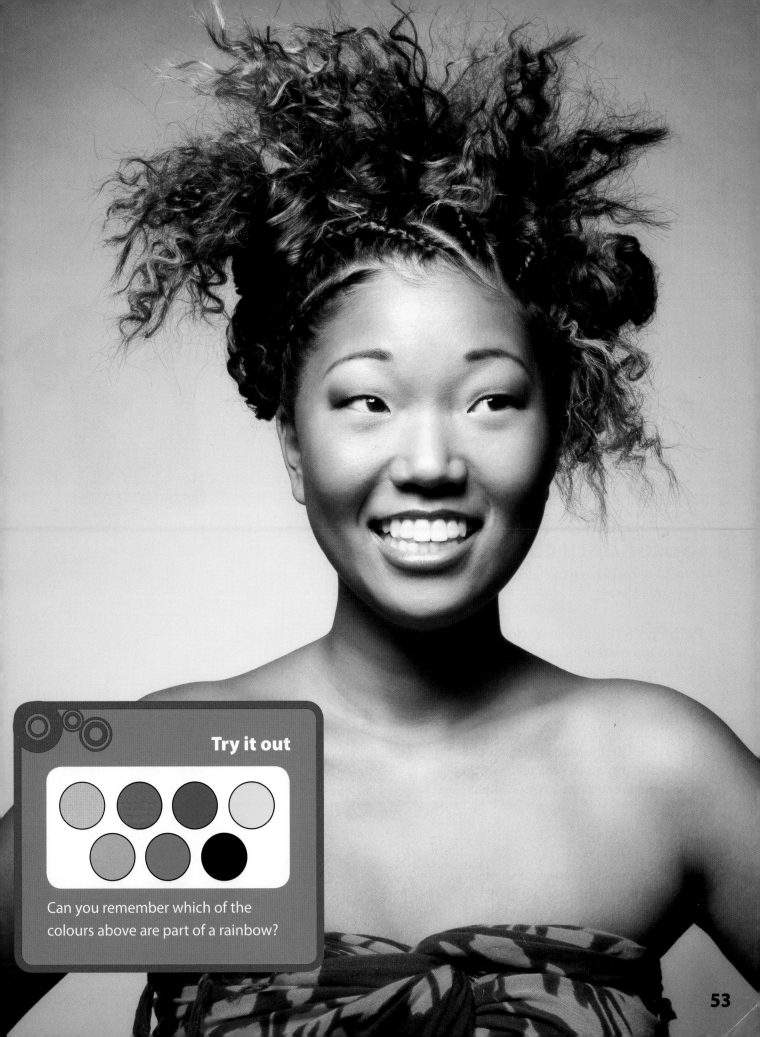

Try it out

Can you remember which of the colours above are part of a rainbow?

53

Knowing the colour spectrum

In this topic you will learn about:

- Primary colours
- Secondary colours
- Colours that cancel each other out (or neutralise)

Q What do you think of the colours on this T-shirt? Do you think they look good together?

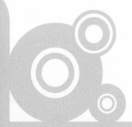

Primary colours.

The primary colours are:

Secondary colours

The secondary colours are made by mixing TWO of the primary colours.

When you take the primary colour **RED**…
…and add the primary colour **YELLOW**…
…you get the secondary colour **ORANGE**.

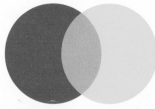

When you take the primary colour **BLUE**…
…and add the primary colour **YELLOW**…
…you get the secondary colour **GREEN**.

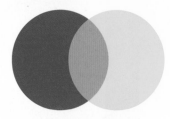

When you take the primary colour **RED**…
…and add the primary colour **BLUE**…
…you get the secondary colour **VIOLET**.

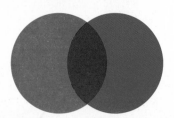

Key term

Violet – another name for purple

Try it out

Mix together red and yellow paint to see what colour you get. Now try adding more red and see if the colour changes.

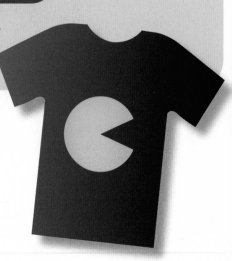

Using colours to cancel each other out

Colours that are opposite each other on the colour star (see right) can be used to cancel each other out (neutralise the colour).
For example:

red **and** green

blue **and** orange

yellow **and** violet

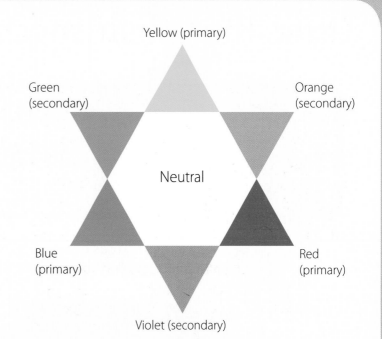

Yellow (primary)

Green (secondary)

Orange (secondary)

Neutral

Blue (primary)

Red (primary)

Violet (secondary)

In the salon

A client came into Lian's salon to have her make-up done – she was going to be a bridesmaid that afternoon. The client was really worried about her cheeks, which always seemed to be red no matter what make-up she tried. Lian told her she would use a green corrective make-up product first. This would neutralise the redness in her cheeks. Then she would apply the wedding make-up on top.
The client was really pleased with the finished look. No red cheeks!

- Why did Lian use a green product?
- Why didn't she use a violet product instead?

Try it out

Apply some blue paint to a piece of paper and then gradually add the orange a little bit at a time. What happens to the blue colour?

Top tip

You can also buy special violet (purple) make-up. This can be used if your skin is sallow. (Sallow means dull and/or yellowish.)

Just checking

1 Which of the following are primary colours?
   a Yellow   **b** Purple   **c** Blue   **d** Green

2 Which of the following are secondary colours?
   a Yellow   **b** Orange   **c** Red   **d** Violet

3 Which colour would you use to cancel out yellow?
   a Green   **b** Blue   **c** Red   **d** Violet

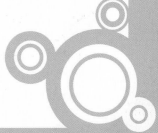

Using the colour spectrum

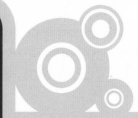

In this topic you will learn about:

- How to use the colour spectrum in the hair and beauty industry to create an image

Q **Look at the images below. Which person do you think has the right hair and make-up colours for their skin tone? Why do you think that?**

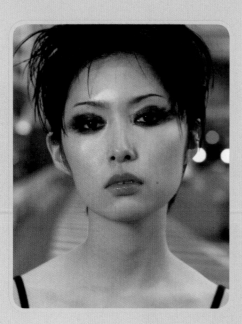 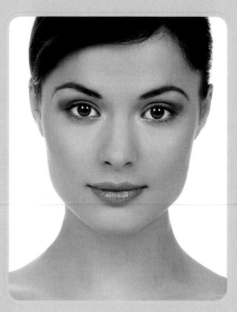

Skin tones

Your skin tone will help you to decide which colours to wear. It will also help you to choose the right colour make-up and hair to suit your skin.

When you are choosing make-up, you need to know if your skin tone is warm or cool. Generally your skin tone will either have pink or yellow **undertones**. You will often hear these skin tones called warm or cool; warm are the yellow tones and cool are the pink/red tones.

If you work with the correct colours for your skin, your make-up will always look better.

Cool

Cool undertones are a combination of reds and blues and generally go with skin tones that are rosy-pink, rosy-beige or dark brown.

Women with cool undertones usually have blue, green or black eyes.

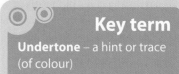

Key term

Undertone – a hint or trace (of colour)

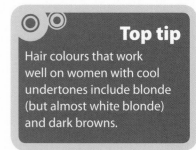

Top tip

Hair colours that work well on women with cool undertones include blonde (but almost white blonde) and dark browns.

Warm

Warm undertones are more yellow and go with skin tones of peach, golden brown, beige, copper or deep golden brown.

Usually women with warm undertones have hazel, brown or **amber** coloured eyes.

In the salon

Navin had an appointment with a client who had naturally dark hair and warm skin tones. The client wanted a completely new look and she asked for white-blonde hair. Navin said it wasn't a good idea with her natural hair colour and skin tones. He suggested a warm copper colour instead. The client wasn't happy as this wasn't what she wanted.

She decided to go to another salon where the stylists were happy to colour her hair white blonde. When the client saw the finished result she was really upset. The colour didn't look the way she thought it would – it made her look ill!

- What do you think went wrong? Was the other salon right to do something that didn't suit the client?

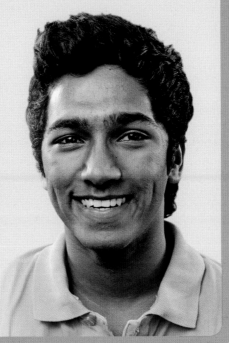

Top tip

Hair colours that work well with warm skin tones are golden brown, chestnut and copper.

Try it out

Are you warm or cool? For true results, you should carry out this test while you're *not* wearing any make-up. Get a piece of silver paper and a piece of gold paper. Hold the silver paper next to your face and see how your skin looks. Then do the same with the gold paper and see which one looks better. If your skin looks glowing and any imperfections seem to disappear (for example, spots), this will be the right one for you. So if your skin looks better next to the silver paper it means you have 'cool' skin tones. If your skin looks better next to the gold paper, you have 'warm' skin tones.

Just checking

1 If you have cool skin tones your eyes may be:
   a Blue
   b Brown
   c Green
   d Hazel

2 You should make sure your hair colour complements your skin tones as this will:
   a Make sure you look poorly all the time
   b Make you look better
   c Make sure you can always wear black clothes
   d Make sure you have lots of friends.

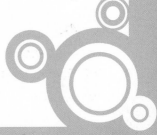

Anatomy and physiology

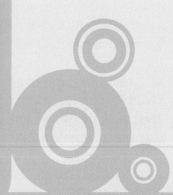

In this unit you will learn about:

- The structure of hair
- Head and face shapes and features
- Body shape
- Hair texture, length, density and elasticity
- Different hair types and hair growth
- Contra-indications to hairdressing services
- The functions of the skin and different skin types
- The bone structure of the face and skull
- The structure of the nail and its functions
- Contra-indications to beauty treatments

Introduction

This section contains all the essential **anatomy** and **physiology** that you will need to be able to assist with and carry out hair and beauty services and treatments.

As an assistant beauty therapist or hairdresser, it is essential that you have a good knowledge of anatomy and physiology. This is because many of the treatments and services that you are learning about will have an effect on the body. For example, a beauty therapist needs to know the effects of massage on circulation, the muscles and the appearance of the skin. As a hairdresser, you need to know about the effects that styling and the use of chemicals will have on the structure of the hair.

Key terms

Anatomy – the framework and structure of the bones and muscles

Physiology – bodily processes

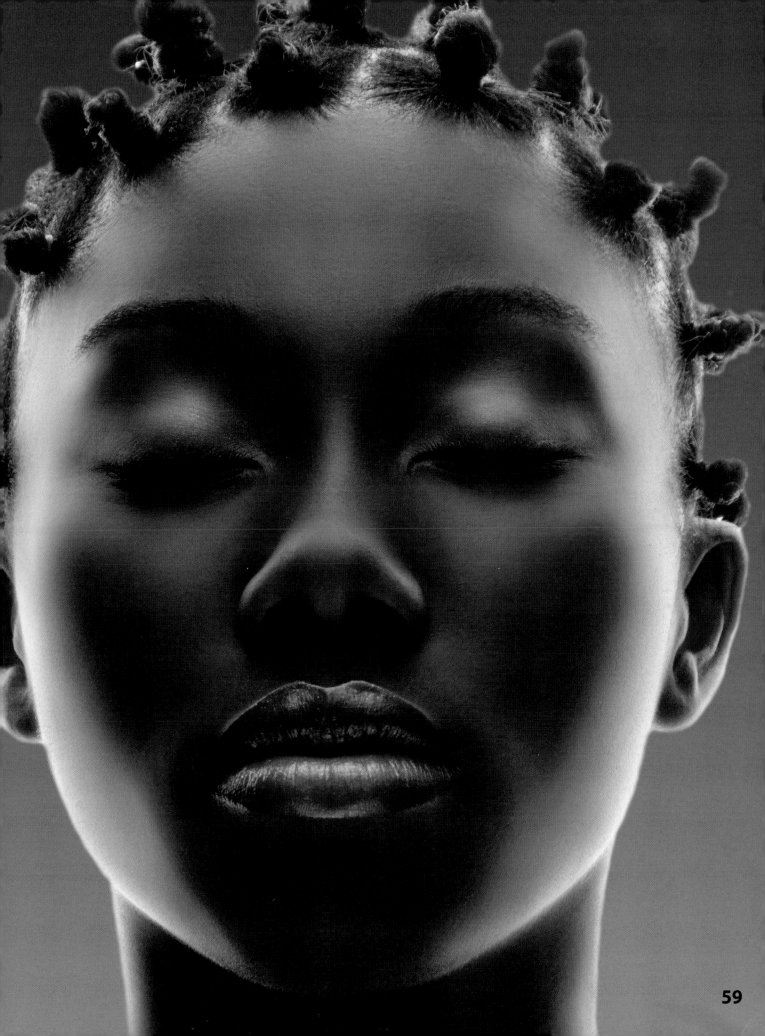

Hair structure and head and face shapes

In this topic you will learn about:

- The hair structure
- Head and face shapes

Q Why do you think it is important to make sure your hairstyle suits your face shape?

Hair structure

You need to understand how hair is made up and how this may affect the hairdressing services you are going to carry out.

The hair has three layers.

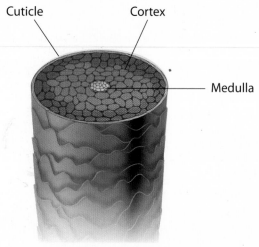

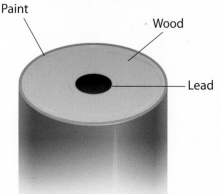

The three layers of the hair – they are a bit like the three parts of a pencil

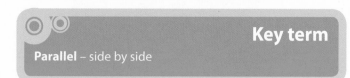

Key term

Parallel – side by side

Try it out

Hold a few strands of your hair near to the roots. Now run your fingers down the hair from the roots to the ends. How does your hair feel? If it feels silky smooth all the way down, it means your cuticles are healthy. But if your hair feels rough and prickly, it means your cuticles are damaged.

The outside layer of the hair is called the cuticle. It is made up from layers of overlapping bands that look a bit like fish scales.

The cuticle protects the inside parts of the hair, but it can be damaged by harsh treatment – for example, having too many colours on the hair or not using straightening irons properly.

The cortex is the next layer. It makes up the largest part of the hair. It is made up from lots of bunches of **parallel** fibres, a bit like holding a handful of drinking straws. This part of the hair is important because it is where the colouring, perming and relaxing processes take place.

The medulla is in the centre of the hair. It is made up of small cells with air spaces in between. It does not affect any of the hairdressing services – in fact some people don't even have one!

Head and face shapes

The shape of the head and face is determined by the way the bones fit together. The ideal face shape is oval and nearly every hairstyle will suit it. Do you know what your face shape is?

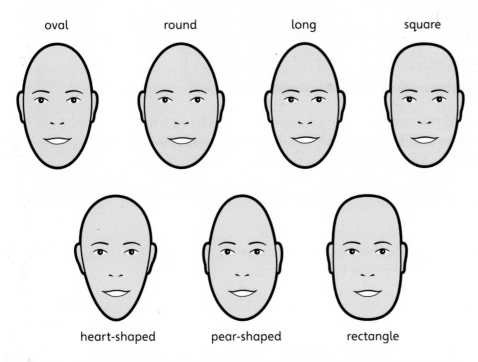

oval   round   long   square

heart-shaped   pear-shaped   rectangle

Different face shapes

Your hair acts as a frame for your face, like a frame around a photograph. The right hairstyle can change the way your face looks and also help to hide any parts of your face that are not quite perfect.

The perfect head **profile** should look like a question mark. With careful styling you can create the **illusion** of a question mark-shaped head! Your hairstyle should also **complement** your body shape. For example, if you are **petite**, avoid a large hairstyle as this will make your body look **out of proportion**.

Just checking

1 The outside layer of the hair is called:
   a The medulla
   b The cuticle
   c The cortex
   d The matrix.

2 What is the ideal face shape?
   a Square
   b Round
   c Oval
   d Heart-shaped

Hair features

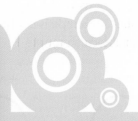

In this topic you will learn about:

- Hair texture, density, length and elasticity

Q Have you ever wondered why some people seem to have a lot of hair and others don't? If you look at different people's hair in ponytails, why do some of them have thick ponytails while others have thin ones?

The topics listed above are things you should consider before carrying out styling services on the hair (including plaiting). If you think about each one, and how it will affect the way you style the hair, you will get the best results.

Hair texture

Hair texture describes how thick or thin each individual strand of hair is. It is important to remember that the texture of someone's hair can vary across the head.

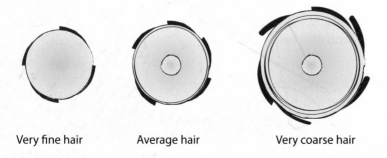

| Very fine hair | Average hair | Very coarse hair |

Try it out

Pull out a hair (or find a loose one on your clothing). Ask some friends to do the same. Compare everyone's hair to see whose is the finest. (You can see the hairs better if you place them on a piece of white paper.)

The texture of the hair will help you to decide which styling products will be most suitable. You can also choose the right size of brush to get the best result if you are blow-drying.

Hair density

Density refers to how much hair someone has. If you put the hair into a ponytail, is it a thick ponytail or a thin one? If it is thick, it means the client's hair is dense. The density of the hair will help you to decide which styling products are most suitable for it. It will also help you to choose a style that will work with that amount of hair.

Hair length

You should always look at the length of the client's hair before you start a shampooing or styling service. It will help you to decide how much product you need to use, for example, how much shampoo. It will also help you to work out if you can get the right style with the client's hair. Sometimes the client's hair is too short for the style they want. At other times it may be too long and heavy and the style won't work.

Hair elasticity

Hair that is in good condition should stretch when it is pulled, but when you stop pulling, it should go back to its original length.

However, if the elasticity is not good, the hair won't return to its original length – it will stay in the stretched state (a bit like an old elastic band). Hair with poor elasticity tells you that the cortex is damaged.

The elasticity of the hair is important when you are styling it. If it is poor, you will not get good results and the hair is often difficult to work with.

Top tip

Make sure you remember the difference between hair texture and hair density. Lots of people confuse the two but they are different. Hair texture refers to the thickness of each strand of hair. Density is how thick or thin the ponytail is.

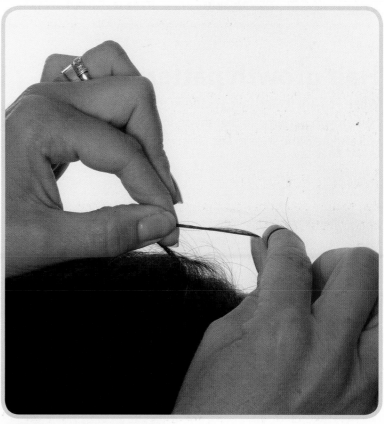

Checking hair elasticity

Just checking

1 Hair density means:
   a How big the client's ponytail will be
   b How big each strand of hair is
   c The growth patterns on the crown
   d The hair will stretch but won't return to its original length.

2 Hair with good elasticity will:
   a Stretch but won't return to its original length
   b Not stretch at all
   c Stretch and return to its original length
   d Need extra products when you're styling the hair.

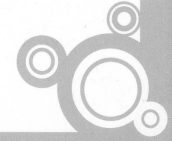

Hair growth patterns

In this topic you will learn about:

- Hair growth patterns

Q **Have you ever wondered why some people's hair sticks up on the crown? Why do you think this is?**

Hair growth patterns

When you are styling hair, you need to work with the hair growth patterns so that the style will lie properly. It will also help the style to last longer!

Try it out

Work with a friend and look at each other's hair at different parts of the head. Look at the front hairline, on the top and in the nape (the back of the head, near the neck). What differences can you see?

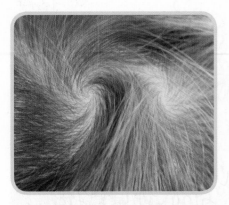

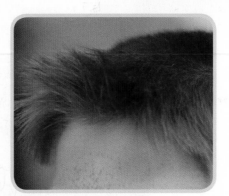

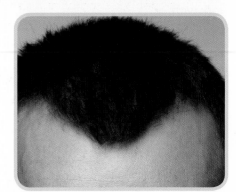

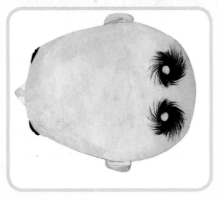

Double crown

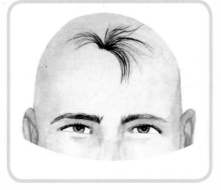

Cowlick

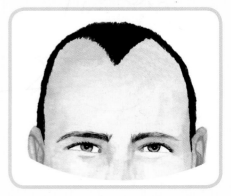

Widow's peak

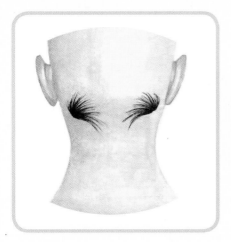
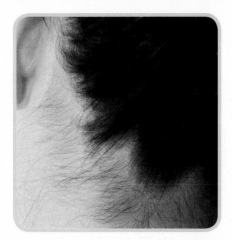

Nape whorl

In the salon

Keeley was asked to carry out a blow-dry on a client with short hair. The client wanted the back of her hair to lie flat and straight. This seemed like an easy task. Keeley started to blow-dry the client's hair but she just couldn't make it lie flat – it kept sticking out. Eventually Keeley went to speak to one of the senior stylists. They pointed out that the client had strong nape whorls. This was why Keeley was finding the blow-dry so difficult. The senior stylist showed Keeley how to work with the nape whorl and dry the hair flat.

- Was Keeley right to ask for help?
- What would you have done in that situation?

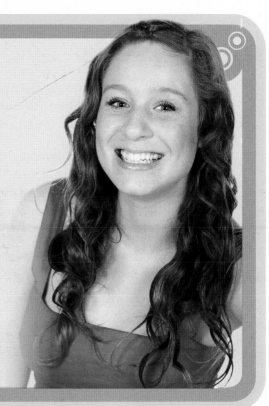

Just checking

1 You would find a cowlick:
   - a   on the front hairline
   - b   in the nape of the neck
   - c   on the crown
   - d   over the ears.

2 Why is it important to work with hair growth patterns when styling hair?
   - a   So you can use a different type of brush
   - b   To make plaits stand out from the head
   - c   To help the styling last longer
   - d   To make sure a nape whorl changes to a double crown

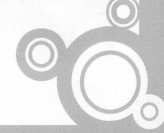

Top tip

If someone has a strong cowlick, it is very difficult to make their fringe lie flat.

Hair types and the hair growth cycle

Q

Have you ever wondered why you have loose hairs in your hairbrush?

Hair types

Hair will usually fall into the following three categories: straight, wavy or curly. Some people's hair may be a mixture. For example, the hair may be very tightly curled with one or two areas where the hair is just wavy.

Hair can also fall into one of the following types:
- Asian/Oriental – hair is usually straight and may be **coarse**.
- Caucasian/European – hair can be straight, wavy or curly.
- African type – hair is curly and the amount of curl can range from very tight curls to loose curls.

If we took a **cross section**, the shape of the hair will be different depending on the hair type.

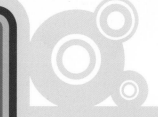

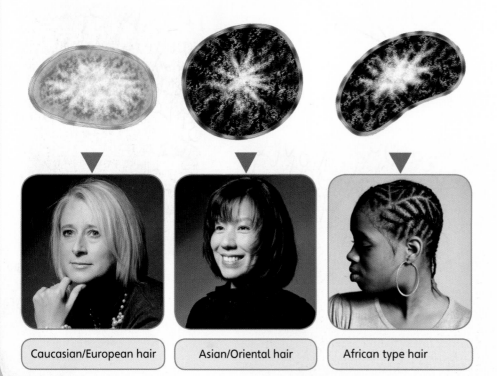

| Caucasian/European hair | Asian/Oriental hair | African type hair |

The hair growth cycle

Hair grows about 1.25 cm each month and each day we lose between 80 and 100 hairs. Each one of the hairs on your head isn't growing all the time. It will grow for a few years, then have a rest and then a new hair starts growing. When the new hair starts to grow, it pushes the old hair out.

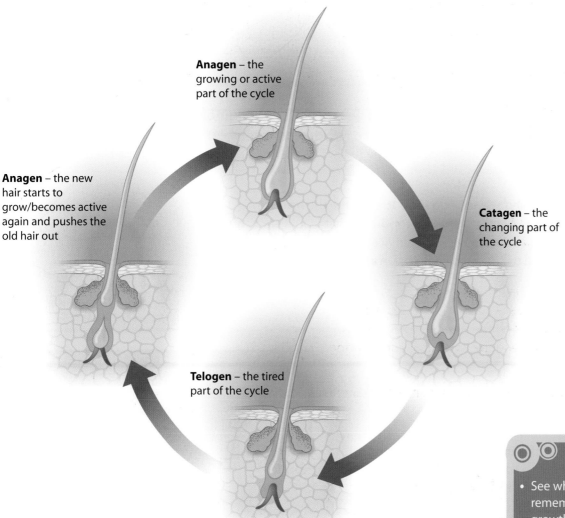

Anagen – the growing or active part of the cycle

Anagen – the new hair starts to grow/becomes active again and pushes the old hair out

Catagen – the changing part of the cycle

Telogen – the tired part of the cycle

Try it out

- See what you can remember about the hair growth cycle. Write your thoughts on a piece of paper then check the book to see how you did.

Functional skills
English reading and writing

Just checking

1 You can identify African type hair because it is:
   a Straight
   b Curly
   c Wavy
   d A mixture of wavy and straight.

2 The active or growing part of the hair growth cycle is called:
   a Telogen
   b Catagen
   c Anagen
   d Melogen.

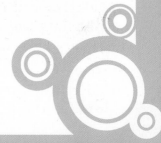

Hairdressing – contra-indications

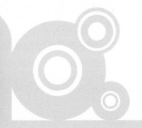

In this topic you will learn about:

- Hair conditions
- Skin and scalp conditions

Q Can you think of something wrong with your hair or skin that might stop you from having a hairdressing service?

Before starting any hairdressing service, you need to examine the hair, skin and scalp. This is because the client may have a **condition** that would stop you from carrying out the service. Alternatively, the service could still be done, but with extreme care. You need to know which hair, skin and scalp conditions will **contra-indicate** the service.

Key terms

Condition – medical problem

Contra-indicate – a reason why something shouldn't be done

Hair conditions

While you are chatting to the client, look at their hair and scalp. Do this discreetly so the client thinks you are just feeling their hair.

Head lice

Head lice are usually found in the nape of the neck or behind the ears, but you should check all over the head just in case. If you find the client has lice or nits, tell your tutor or manager immediately (but discreetly). The client will not be able to have the service until the head lice have been treated.

Skin and scalp conditions

As well as looking for head lice, you must make sure the skin and scalp are suitable for the hairdressing service.

Sometimes clients have areas on their skin or scalp that are red and swollen. This would usually be because they have an infection (or the beginning of one) or because they have a skin disorder such as eczema, in which case it may be sore.

If a client has open cuts or scratches on their scalp, products may get into them, causing pain and discomfort. There is also the risk of a cut becoming infected.

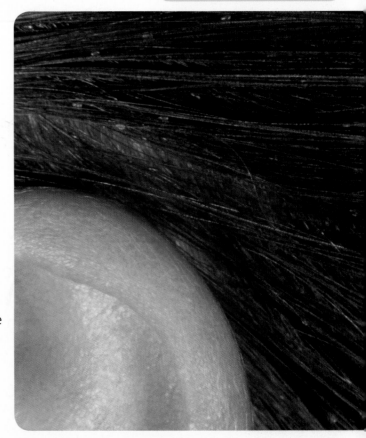

Here you can see the eggs (nits) laid by head lice

Skin condition		Description
Eczema	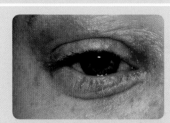	There may be patches of dry skin which can itch, become sore and weep. It might not stop you carrying out the service, unless the skin is broken; for example, it is weeping fluid.
Psoriasis	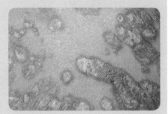	You may notice red areas on the scalp that are covered with silvery scales. It shouldn't stop you from carrying out the service unless the client has scratched the skin until it has bled.
Impetigo	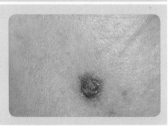	If the skin or scalp is red and swollen, look closely to see if there is any pus (it will be yellow, like really bad spots). It could mean the client has a bacterial infection which could then be passed on to other people. An example of this would be the skin condition impetigo.
Dandruff	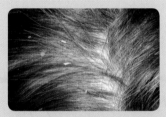	You also need to check the client's scalp for dandruff. You can help them with this condition by using an anti-dandruff shampoo.
Contact dermatitis	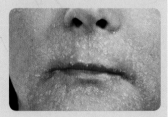	Contact dermatitis is the most common type of dermatitis. It means that the skin has come into contact with something that has irritated it. This might be shampoo, hair colour or cleaning products. A lot of hairdressers have to give up hairdressing if they develop dermatitis.

Just checking

1 It is important to check the client's hair, skin and scalp before a hairdressing service:
   a So you look important
   b To avoid cross-infection
   c To make sure the hair is clean
   d So your boss will think you're clever.

2 Impetigo is a bacterial infection. You can tell this because:
   a The area will look clear
   b The client has a very flaky scalp
   c The skin will look red
   d The area will have big yellow spots.

Try it out

Use textbooks or the Internet to see if you can find any other hair and scalp conditions. Write down your answers and ask your tutor to check them.

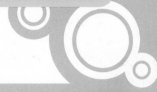 **Functional skills**
English writing, ICT

The structure and functions of the skin

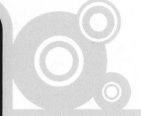

In this topic you will learn about:

- The structure and functions of the skin
- Factors affecting skin type

Q The skin is the largest organ of the body and is airtight and watertight. Do you know the average weight of an adult human's skin?

The structure of the skin

The skin is made up of three layers:

- Epidermis – this is made up of five different layers and the only one you can see is the outer layer. It is this that you apply skin care and make-up products to.
- The dermis – this is the more sensitive layer of the skin and contains nerve endings, sweat and sebaceous glands, and blood and lymph vessels.
- The subcutaneous layer – this is the fatty layer.

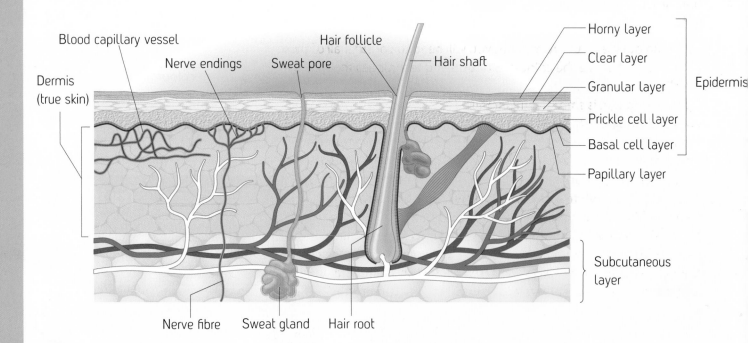

The basic structure of the skin

The functions of the skin

The skin does many important jobs. Without it, our bodies could overheat, become ill and get injured easily.

- Vitamin production – the sun's rays on the skin make vitamin D (essential for strong bones and teeth).
- Sense and feeling – the nerve endings in our skin are very sensitive. They pick up changes in temperature or pressure, and alert us to pain.
- Heat control – skin helps to control the temperature in our body. When we are too hot, we begin to sweat and this cools us down. When we are too cold, we begin to shiver, which warms up the body.
- Absorption – the skin is able to absorb small amounts of products that are put on the skin.
- Protection – skin is like a waterproof jacket. It provides the body with protection from dirt, bacteria and injury.
- Excretion – some waste products and toxins are removed from the body through our sweat.
- Secretion – the skin produces a substance through its pores called sebum. It keeps our skin smooth and supple and free from splits and cracks that would let in germs.
- Storage – the skin stores fat and water. Without them we could not survive.

Factors affecting skin type

Skin type and characteristics such as colouring and condition vary between people. The type and characteristics depend on:

- age
- ethnic group
- gender.

When carrying out make-up treatments, you will need to consider all of these things. They will influence the colours, products and techniques that you will use on a client.

- Age – young skin is smooth and blemish-free whereas mature skin has lines and wrinkles. This makes make-up more difficult to apply.
- Ethnic group – different coloured skin means you will have to consider the colours that you use to complement it. For example, it would not be suitable to apply a dark foundation colour to a light Caucasian skin.
- Caucasian skin is white and comes mostly from European origins.
- Oriental skin has a yellowish tone and is oily.
- Asian skin has a medium to dark tone with yellow base colour.
- African-Caribbean skin is dark and ranges in colour to almost black.
- Gender – female skin tends to be more sensitive and thinner than male skin, so more care will need to be taken when applying make-up.

Just checking

1 How many layers does the epidermis have?

2 Where would you find the nerve endings?

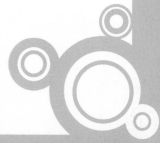

Skin types and conditions

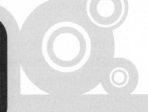

Q **Would you use the same products on every client? If not, why not?**

Skin types and conditions

Normal skin is not often found in adults. It is usually found in children and young people. This type of skin needs lots of gentle care to keep it normal.

Oily skin is caused when too much oil is produced in the skin. We need oil to keep the skin smooth but when the skin produces too much it causes problems. An oily skin can start or become worse as a teenager during puberty.

Dry skin lacks oil because the oil glands in the skin do not produce enough. It must be moisturised well. Poor diet and not drinking enough water can cause dry skin or make it worse.

Combination skin is made up of two skin types. These types vary, but the most common is normal or dry skin on the cheek area, and an oily part on the nose and chin, and across the forehead (known as the T-zone). The oily T-zone shows up as a shiny nose, chin and forehead with blackheads.

Try it out

- In small groups, try to identify the skin types of your classmates. Think about how to recognise the different types. You might need to ask each other questions to find out more.

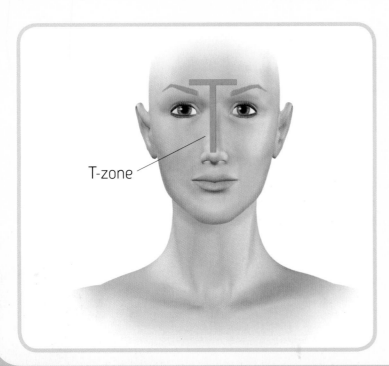

T-zone

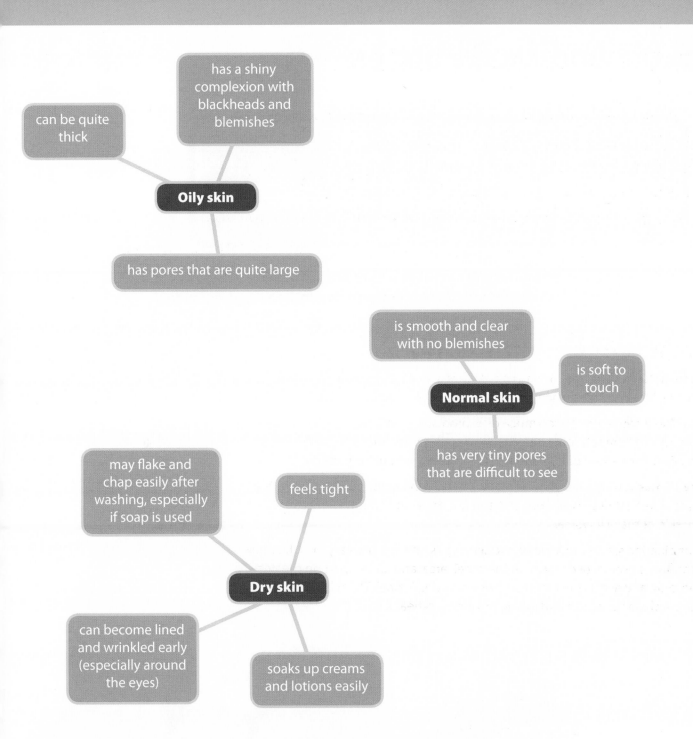

has a shiny complexion with blackheads and blemishes

can be quite thick

Oily skin

has pores that are quite large

is smooth and clear with no blemishes

is soft to touch

Normal skin

has very tiny pores that are difficult to see

may flake and chap easily after washing, especially if soap is used

feels tight

Dry skin

can become lined and wrinkled early (especially around the eyes)

soaks up creams and lotions easily

Just checking

1 State the four main skin types.

2 State the four main ethnic skin colours.

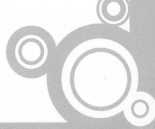

Skull and facial bones

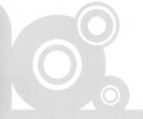

In this topic you will learn about:

- The bones of the skull
- The bones of the face

Q **Did you know that when we are born, our bones are softer and less strong and they harden and strengthen as we get older?**

The skull

The bones of the head, known as the skull, keep the muscles in place and protect the brain and other parts of the head from injury. The skull is made up of the cranium and the lower jaw (mandible). There are 22 bones in the skull. Eight of these are in the cranium, as shown in the table below.

Bone	Position
1 x ethmoid bone	At the roof of the nose
1 x frontal bone	Forms the front of the cranium, forehead and upper eye sockets
1 x occipital bone	At the back and lower part of the cranium
2 x parietal bones	At the back and top of the cranium
1 x sphenoid bone	At the base of the cranium, in front of the temporal bones
2 x temporal bones	At the side, around the ears

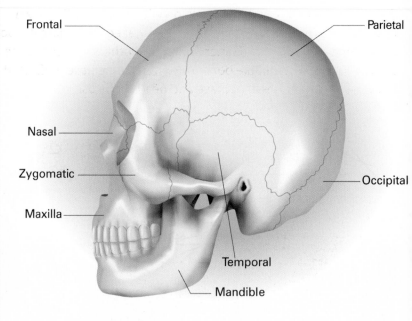

The bones of the skull

The face

The bones of the face also protect the soft tissues inside the head. The face is made up of 14 bones. The seven main ones are shown in the table below.

Bone	Position
1 x mandible	This is the lower jaw and is the only moving bone in the face. It enables the mouth to move for chewing and talking.
2 x maxillae	These form the upper jaw, most of the side wall of the nose and the front part of the soft palate (the top of the mouth).
2 x nasal bones	These form the bridge (upper part) of the nose.
2 x zygomatic bones	These form the cheekbones.

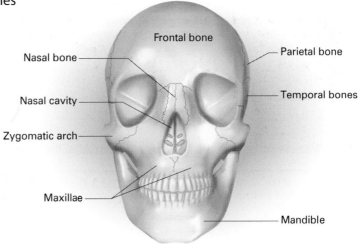

The bones of the face

How the bones affect facial shape

The photograph below shows a person with prominent (noticeable) cheekbones. The bones that create this are called the zygomatic bones and some people have less prominent ones than others. The line of the chin and jaw is affected by the mandible bone. The shape of the nose is affected by the nasal bones. All of the bones in our face and head shape us.

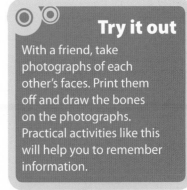

Try it out

With a friend, take photographs of each other's faces. Print them off and draw the bones on the photographs. Practical activities like this will help you to remember information.

Just checking

1 How many bones are there in the face?
   a 5
   b 8
   c 14
   d 22

2 Which bone might you apply cheek colour to?
   a Maxilla
   b Mandible
   c Zygomatic
   d Occipital

3 Name one function of bone.

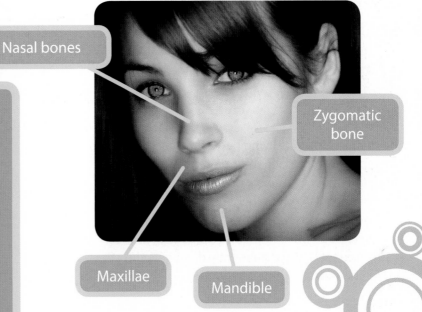

Nasal bones

Zygomatic bone

Maxillae

Mandible

The bones of the face affect its shape

The nails

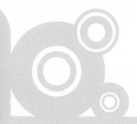

In this topic you will learn about:
- The structure of the nail
- The parts and functions of the nail

Q **What do you think nails are made of? What is the thing that makes them hard?**

It is useful to understand the structure of the hand and nails when you are carrying out nail treatments. Clients might appreciate this information too because it will help them to keep their hands and nails healthy.

The structure of nails

The nails grow from the ends of the fingers and toes. The nail plate is a hard, rectangular and curved structure. It covers and protects the sensitive fingertips and nail bed. When healthy, a nail should be pink, smooth and flexible with a white free edge that shows no signs of flaking or splitting. The cuticle should not be dry, rough or inflamed.

Parts and functions of the nail

Matrix

The matrix is the only living part of the nail. It produces and replaces the cells that form the nail. The nail's condition depends on how healthy the cell growth is and whether or not there has been any damage to the matrix. Damage could be caused by injury, poor treatment or an infection. However, as long as the matrix has not been permanently damaged, the effect on the nail is usually only temporary.

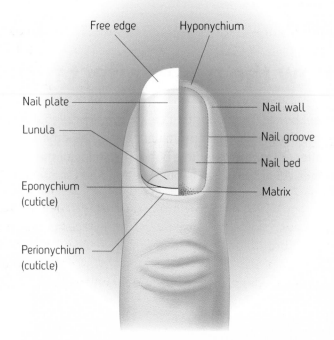

The structure of the nail unit

Lunula

The lunula is also known as the half moon. It is found on all nails, but it is easier to see on some than on others. It is at the base of the nails and is the part of the matrix you can see.

Nail bed

The nail bed is the healthy soft tissue underneath the nail plate. It gives the nail its pink appearance. It contains blood vessels and nerve endings. Ridges in the nail bed help to keep the nail firmly in place as it grows.

Nail plate

The nail plate lies on top of the nail bed and is the main part of the nail. It is pink because of the soft tissue which you can see underneath. The nail plate is made up of layers of fat, moisture and growth cells, and these give the nail its strength. If you tear part of the nail off, it is very painful because it is attached to blood vessels and nerve endings.

Free edge

The free edge is the hardest part of the nail. It grows past the end of the nail bed and fingertip. It is whitish in colour. This is because it has grown beyond the pink tissue. It does not hurt if you break it because it is not joined to blood vessels or nerve endings.

Nail grooves or nail wall

The nail grooves are deep ridges that lie along the back and sides of the nail. The grooves at the side of the nail guide the direction of the nail growth. The grooves also help to stop germs getting into the nail bed. Hangnails can appear if the nail grooves are not kept soft and well moisturised. These are dry strips of skin at the sides of the nail that can become very sore and inflamed if left untreated or pulled off.

Cuticle

The cuticle is at the base of the nail. It protects the matrix from germs by forming a barrier. You should never cut the cuticle off during a manicure. If you do, the matrix could become infected.

Perionychium (cuticle) Eponychium (cuticle) Nail plate Free edge Nail fold Matrix Nail bed Hyponychium

Try it out

In groups you are going to make a pack of cards. Each card will have a nail part on one side and a description on the other. Each person in the group must choose a part of the nail and make their card. These key cards can be used to revise the structure of the nails.

Just checking

1 What is the function of the nail grooves?

2 What is the nail plate made up of?

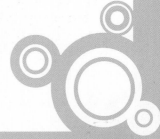

Contra-indications for a facial treatment

In this topic you will learn about:
- Skin conditions

Q **Can you think of something that might stop you from having a facial treatment?**

Before treating a client, you need to examine the skin (if you're working on the face) or the nails and skin surrounding them (if you're carrying out a manicure, pedicure or any other nail treatment). This is because the client may have a **condition** that may stop the treatment from going ahead.

The things you should look for before carrying out a treatment on the face are shown in this spider diagram (right): All of these could **contra-indicate** a facial treatment.

Condition		Description
Cold sores	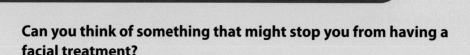	These are usually found on the lips and underneath the nose. They are an infection caused by a virus and can be passed from one person to another easily.
Eye infection – conjunctivitis		The eye looks red and watery and is often sore and itchy. It can be caused by various things such as an allergy.
Scar tissue		If the scar tissue is less than 6 months old you should be very careful when working around the scar or avoid the area altogether.
Eczema		The skin is very dry and often flaky. It can sometimes be red, itchy and very sore for the client. You may need to avoid this area as it could make the eczema worse.

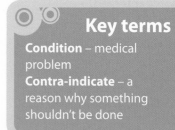

Key terms

Condition – medical problem

Contra-indicate – a reason why something shouldn't be done

When carrying out any treatment where you are working on the nails and surrounding areas, you should be looking for the things shown in the spider diagram (below):

Try it out

Using a magnifying lamp, study the skin of one of your classmates more closely. See what you can find that wasn't visible to the naked eye.

Redness – this may be an allergy, sunburn or an injury

Blisters around the mouth and nose – this may be a cold sore

Bloodshot and watery eyes – this may be an eye infection

Things you should look for before a facial treatment

Swelling – this could be bruising or something more serious

Dry, red, flaky skin – this may be eczema or dermatitis

Scar tissue

Cuts and abrasions

Just checking

1 If a client had patches of eczema on her eyelids, what would you do?
   a Try to avoid the eye area, but apply make-up to the rest of her face
   b Tell the client she can't have the service done
   c Apply make-up to the client's eyes, but not to the rest of her face

2 If the inside of a client's eyes looked bloodshot and weepy, this could indicate:
   a cold sores
   b   conjunctivitis
   c styes
   d eczema

Top tip

Make sure the skin is clean and free from make-up when carrying out your consultation. Contra-indications may be hidden.

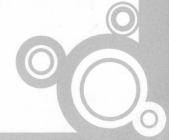

Contra-indications for a manicure/pedicure

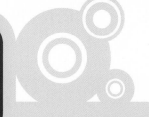

In this topic you will learn about:
- Nail conditions

Q Can you think of something that might stop you from having a beauty treatment?

Condition		Description
Athlete's foot	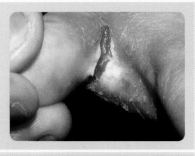	Athlete's foot is also called ringworm of the foot. It is a fungal infection (caused by a fungus) and makes the skin between the toes flake and itch. This can easily be passed from one person to another, so you wouldn't be able to carry out a pedicure on a client with athlete's foot.
Ringworm of the nail (sometimes called onychomycosis)	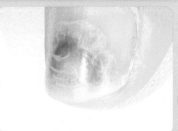	This is also a fungal infection and can affect both toenails and fingernails. The nail plate may look yellow or thickened and the nails can become rough and crumbly.
Verruca (plural = veruccae)	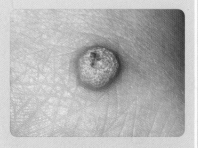	A verruca is a wart on the sole of the foot. Warts normally grow upwards from the surface of the skin but the weight of the body presses it into the foot. This can be very painful. Verrucae can be easily recognised because they have little black dots in them.
Infected 'hangnail' (sometimes called paronychia)	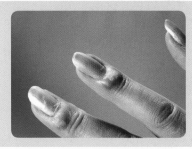	This is an infection of the nail fold. The nail fold is where the nail and skin meet at the sides and base of the nail and this becomes infected. It can affect both the toenails and the fingernails.

You should not carry out a manicure if your client has infected fingernails. Similarly, do not carry out a pedicure if your client's toenails are infected.

You should also check whether your client has any allergies. There may be ingredients in some of the products you use that could cause the client to have an allergic reaction. This is when they itch or sneeze or their skin reddens and maybe even swells. A very bad reaction could mean they have to go to hospital.

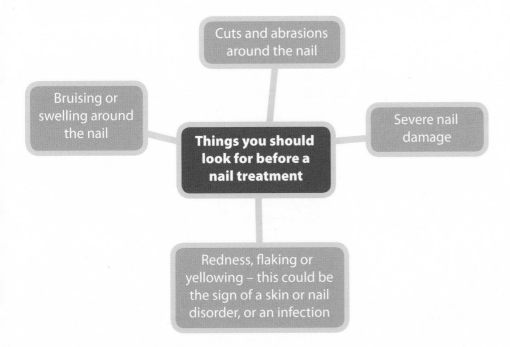

Cuts and abrasions around the nail

Bruising or swelling around the nail

Things you should look for before a nail treatment

Severe nail damage

Redness, flaking or yellowing – this could be the sign of a skin or nail disorder, or an infection

Top tip

If you decide to treat a client with a contra-indication you could make the condition worse or spread infection to others.

Treating contra-indications

Although many contra-indications can be worked around and the treatment adapted, you must check with your tutor or manager first. It is not your responsibility to make the decision about whether or not it is safe to carry on with the treatment.

Try it out

Find clear photographs of disorders and diseases on the Internet. Make large wall posters with the pictures and add brief descriptions underneath them. This will help you start to recognise possible contra-indications that you may see during a consultation and that you need to check out with your tutor.

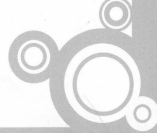
Functional skills
English reading and writing, ICT

Just checking

1 If a client had a minor cut on the skin around the nail, would it be OK to continue with a manicure service?
   a Yes, if the cut was covered up
   b Yes
   c If the client says I can
   d No

2 If a client had athlete's foot, would you be able to carry out a manicure?
   a No
   b Yes
   c Maybe
   d Only if the client could run fast

Shampoo and conditioning

In this unit you will learn about:

- Preparing for shampooing and conditioning hair
- Carrying out a shampoo, condition and towel dry

Introduction

The shampoo and conditioning service is very important in the salon as it prepares the hair for the next part of the service, for example, blow-drying. If the shampooing and conditioning service is carried out well, it puts the client in a good mood – if not, the client may get bad tempered!

You will learn how to prepare the client for the shampoo and conditioning service and which products you should use to get the best results. You will also learn about different massage techniques and when to use them. You will show you can do this by carrying out a shampooing and conditioning service in a safe and hygienic way, followed by towel drying the hair.

Top tip

If you use the right shampoo and conditioning products, you will get the best results. Try to learn about the different shampoos and conditioners in your salon.

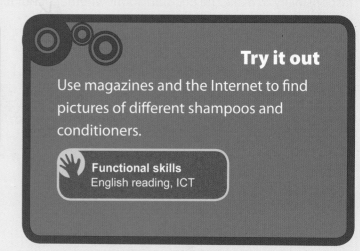

Try it out

Use magazines and the Internet to find pictures of different shampoos and conditioners.

Functional skills
English reading, ICT

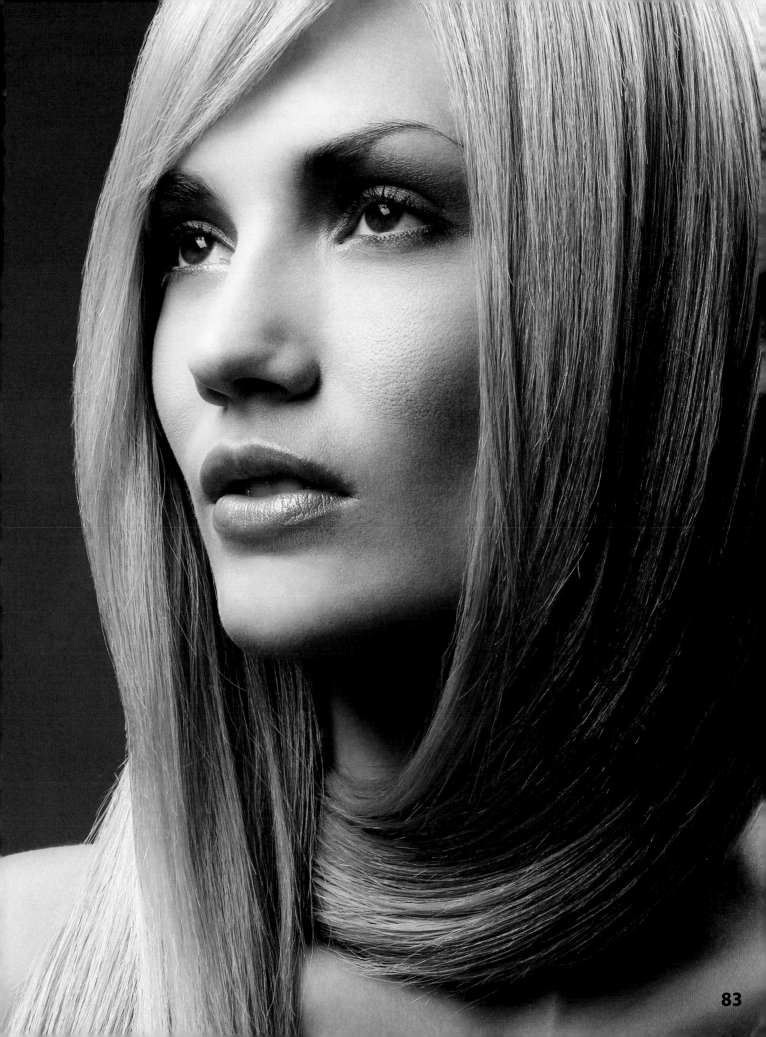

Preparing for shampooing and conditioning

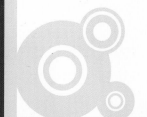

In this topic you will learn about:

- Preparing the client and the importance of using a gown and towel
- Why we shampoo and condition the hair
- Choosing the right products (shampoo and conditioner) for the hair type

Q You will notice that you always wear a gown and a towel when you are having your hair done. Why do you think this is?

Preparing the client

Clients must always wear a clean gown to protect their clothes from spillages. A clean towel around the client's shoulders will also help to protect their clothes from spillages during the shampooing process, and to absorb water and any dripping products.

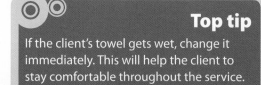

Top tip

If the client's towel gets wet, change it immediately. This will help the client to stay comfortable throughout the service.

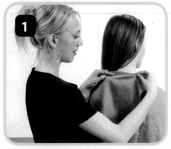

1 Gown the client to protect her clothing.

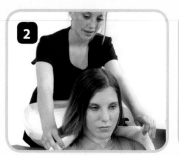

2 Place a towel around the client's shoulders.

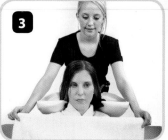

3 Place a towel around the front of the client.

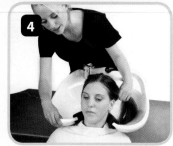

4 Position the client at the basin, making sure she is comfortable.

Why do we use shampoos and conditioners?

Shampoo products are used to make sure the hair and scalp are clean and ready for the next service.

Conditioners close and smooth the cuticle. They add shine and replace moisture in the hair. They also make it easier to **detangle** the hair.

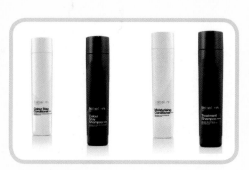

Choosing the correct products, tools and equipment

Before you start to shampoo the hair, you need to know what products, tools and equipment you may need and why you need them.

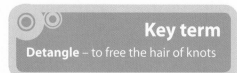

Key term

Detangle – to free the hair of knots

Tools and equipment		Why they are used
Front wash		Used to shampoo hair – some clients may prefer a front wash
Backwash		Used to shampoo the hair, especially good for long hair
Rake comb		Used to detangle the hair

You will need to identify what hair condition each client has.

- Normal hair feels smooth to the touch and generally looks shiny and healthy.
- Dry hair often feels dry and a bit rough to the touch.
- Oily hair is usually oily at the roots. As it is oily, it can often look shiny.
- A dandruff-affected scalp is usually dry and flaky and sometimes it can be itchy.
- Damaged hair looks dull and often feels dry and **brittle**.

Most children have normal hair and when it is brushed it looks silky and smooth. However, because of body changes, most teenagers go through a phase of having oily hair and skin.

It is important to make sure you are using the correct shampoo and conditioning products for the different hair and scalp conditions. You might find it helpful to use a shampooing consultation sheet.

Shampoo Service Consultation Sheet

Student's name _____

Client's name _____

Date _____

Client's hair condition:
- ☐ Dry
- ☐ Normal
- ☐ Oily
- ☐ Dandruff affected

Hair length:
- ☐ Long
- ☐ Medium
- ☐ Short

Has the client's hair been coloured, permed or relaxed?
- ☐ Coloured
- ☐ Permed
- ☐ Relaxed

Which shampoo should be used? _____

Which conditioner should be used? _____

A shampooing consultation sheet

Overuse of chemicals on the hair; for example, hair colour, bleach, relaxer

Reasons why hair may be damaged

Being out in strong sunlight or wind

Incorrect use of heated styling equipment; for example, straightening irons can cause the hair to become **brittle**

Reasons why hair may be damaged

Key term

Brittle – easily broken

Try it out

Look at the different shampoos and conditioners in your salon and find out which products you would use on the following hair and scalp conditions:
- dry hair
- normal hair
- oily hair
- damaged hair
- dandruff-affected scalp

Just checking

1 You must gown the client properly for the shampooing service to:
   a Keep the client warm
   b Keep the boss happy
   c Protect their clothes from spillages
   d Prevent them from breathing in hairspray.

2 You can recognise dry hair because:
   a It feels smooth to the touch and generally looks shiny and healthy
   b It is usually oily at the roots
   c The scalp is usually dry and flaky and sometimes it can be itchy
   d The hair looks dull and often feels dry and brittle.

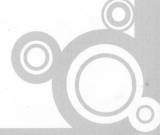

Carry out the shampooing service

In this topic you will learn about:

- Massage techniques when shampooing
- How to shampoo the hair

Q Why do you think it is important to talk to your client in a professional way throughout the shampooing service? What might it feel like for the client if you didn't speak?

Massage techniques for shampooing

Before you start to shampoo the hair you need to know the two different massage movements needed.

Massage movement	Description	
Effleurage	This is the movement used to apply shampoo and conditioner. It is a smooth stroking movement that starts at the front of the head and covers the whole scalp.	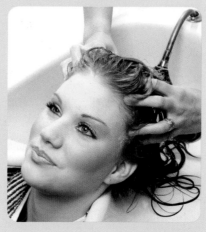
Rotary	This is the rubbing movement you do when you shampoo hair. Rotary should be carried out in a **methodical** way, using the pads of your fingers and working in small round movements over the scalp.	

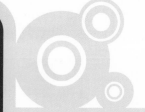

Top tip

Shampooing is very important as it prepares the hair for the next service. If it is done well, the client will feel relaxed and ready to enjoy the rest of their service.

Key term

Methodical – following a pattern

Shampooing the hair

When you are shampooing a client's hair, make sure you have the water temperature and flow right. If there is not enough water, it will take you a long time to rinse off the shampoo and conditioner. If the water is coming out too quickly, it may spray everywhere and wet the client.

You should also check the water temperature before you put it near your client's head. Test the water on the back of your hand or the inside of your wrist. If the temperature feels all right for you, it should be fine for the client, but remember to ask them.

Top tip

If the water is too cold it will shock the client; if too hot it could burn their scalp! Remember to turn the water off while you are shampooing. This will save water and money.

How to shampoo the hair

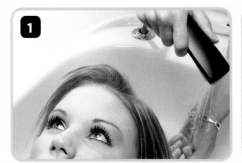

Test the water temperature on the inside of your wrist.

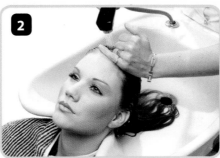

Check the temperature with the client. Thoroughly wet the hair and scalp. Turn off the water.

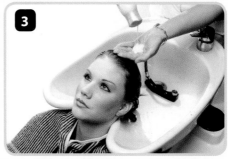

Squeeze a small amount of shampoo into the palm of your hand and smooth between both palms. Apply the shampoo using effleurage.

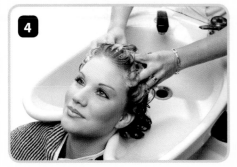

Use rotary massage until the whole head has been covered and the shampoo begins to lather.

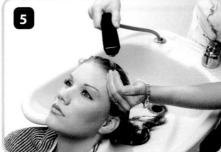

Rinse off the shampoo thoroughly. Now give the client's hair a second shampoo, repeating the process as for the first shampoo. When you have rinsed off the second shampoo, gently squeeze the hair to remove excess water.

Try it out

Have a go at shampooing your friend's hair. Ask them to tell you honestly what they thought of your technique.

Just checking

1 The name of the massage movement you use when you are applying shampoo and conditioner is:
   a Effleurage   b Rotary   c Effleury.

2 When you are shampooing, you should test the water on:
   a The client's head
   b Your upper arm
   c The inside of of your wrist
   d The client's arm.

Carry out the conditioning service

In this topic you will learn about:

- Massage techniques and how to condition the hair
- How to wrap and towel dry the hair
- How to clean and tidy the work area

Q Not everyone uses conditioner. Why do you think this is? Do you think it's important to use conditioner after shampooing the hair?

Massage technique for conditioning

The massage movement you should use when you condition a client's hair is called petrissage. It is quite like rotary, as you still do a methodical massage in small round movements using the pads of your fingers. However, it is a much slower and firmer movement.

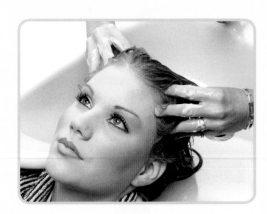

How to condition the hair

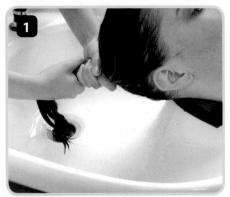

1 After rinsing the shampoo out of the hair, squeeze out all the excess water. (The water should be turned off.)

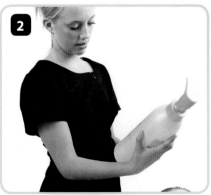

2 Choose the right conditioner for the client.

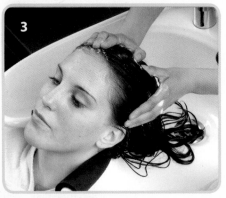

3 Apply the conditioner using the effleurage movement and then massage the scalp using petrissage. Do this for a couple of minutes or following the manufacturer's instructions.

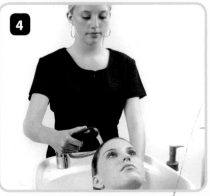

4 Turn on the water. Rinse the hair thoroughly to make sure you remove all the conditioner. If you don't, the hair will look lank and greasy and will be hard to style. Turn off the water.

How to wrap and dry the hair

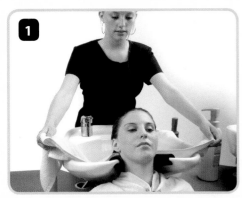

Take a towel and place at the back of the head.

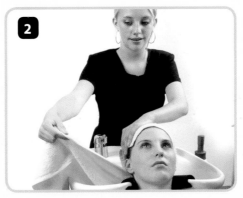

Take one side of the towel across, then the other.

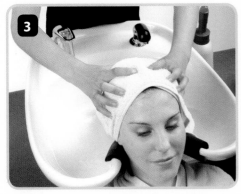

Gently press the towel against the hair to remove excess moisture.

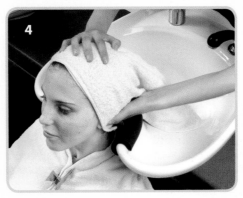

Help the client to sit up.

Clean and tidy the work area

At the end of the service, make sure the basin area is left clean and tidy. The next client will not want to come to a dirty basin, full of someone else's hair and shampoo everywhere. Cleaning also helps to stop cross-infection.

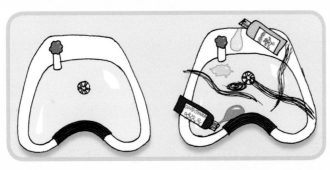

Which basin would you prefer to use?

Just checking

1 Which massage movements are used during the conditioning process?

2 Why is it important to wrap and towel dry the client's hair before you move them to the work station?

3 Why should the basin area be left clean and tidy at the end of the shampooing and conditioning service?

Top tip

Give clients plenty of time when you are helping them to sit up after the shampooing and conditioning service. (Sometimes clients can feel a bit dizzy if they sit up too quickly.) Make sure you are supporting their head while they are sitting up.

Top tip

Reread the section about PPE, COSHH and keeping your equipment clean and sterilised in *Follow health and safety in the salon*, pages 22, 24 and 28–29.

Try it out

Try doing a scalp (petrissage) massage on your friend. If you are applying enough pressure you should see your friend's forehead moving up and down. Don't forget to ask your friend how the massage felt. Feedback from friends and clients will help you to perfect your massage technique.

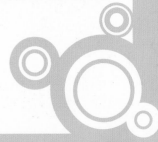

Functional skills
English speaking and listening

Styling women's and men's hair

In this unit you will learn about:

- Products
- Tools and equipment
- Preparing for styling men's and women's hair
- Techniques for styling women's and men's hair including
  - Straightening and smoothing
  - Finger drying
  - Blow-drying
  - Hair up
  - Pin curling
  - Setting

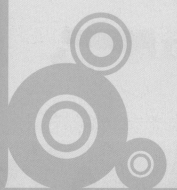

Introduction

The final styling is important because it creates the overall finished look. How many clients would be happy to leave the salon with their hair wet after a cut or colour and go home to dry it themselves? Not many! You must be able to style the hair into a professional finish in order to complete a professional service.

There are different products, tools and equipment available to help you style. You need to become familiar with each and how to use it correctly and to best effect.

Top tips

- Keep some brief notes on the effects of the styling products you use in your salon. Read them often and learn the hairdressing terminology that is used. It will show your clients that you are professional and have good product knowledge.

- Blow-drying is carried out with a variety of brushes but the hair must always be sectioned off into manageable amounts of hair. This makes sure it is controlled properly and dried thoroughly.

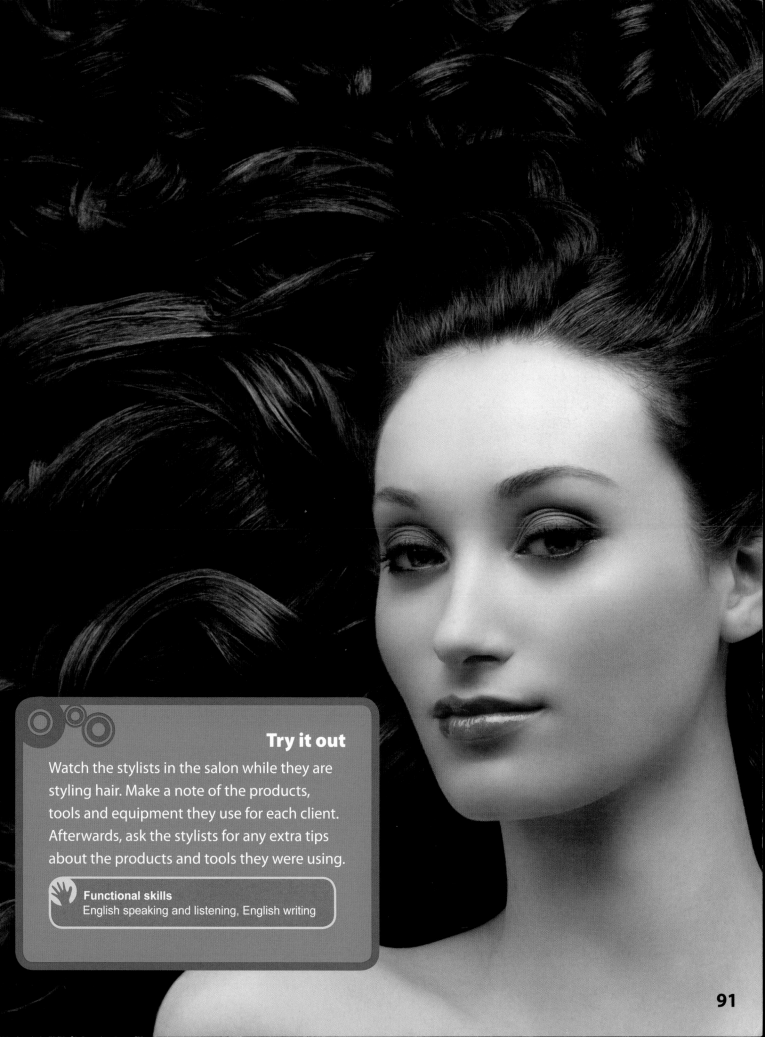

Try it out

Watch the stylists in the salon while they are styling hair. Make a note of the products, tools and equipment they use for each client. Afterwards, ask the stylists for any extra tips about the products and tools they were using.

Functional skills
English speaking and listening, English writing

Products

Do you already have experience of using professional styling products? Do you notice a difference in what you can achieve?

Although men's and women's styling products are packaged differently, they still serve the same purpose (for example, to give hold or add shine).

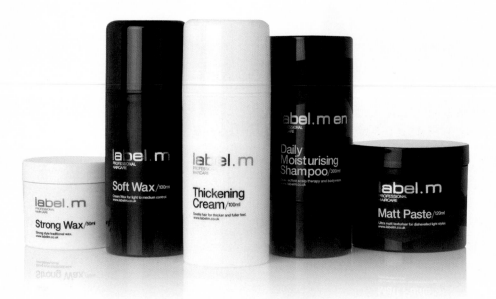

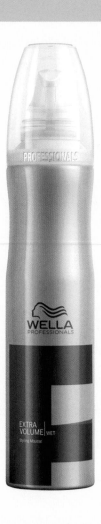

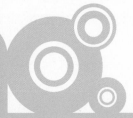

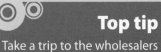

Top tip

Take a trip to the wholesalers and look around at the products, tools and equipment on offer. You may find some inspiration!

Product	Purpose
Mousse	Provides hold and volume to a style, or curl definition if hair is curly
Gel	Provides strong hold to a style. Can dry into the hair or be left for a wet look
Lotion	Provides soft hold to a style for more natural looks
Spray	Holds the style in place after finishing. Helps to beat humidity and reduce static
Moisturisers	Some hold but mainly adds moisture to the hair for very dry or damaged hair
Wax	Soft hold, mainly adds definition and separates curls
Dressing cream	Holds curls and waves in place and good for fine, flyaway hair as prevents static
Heat protector	Helpful when using excessive heat – for example, straightening irons or curling tongs – to help protect the hair from heat damage

In the salon

Jacob was just finishing styling his last client, who was also his good friend. They were going out that evening and Jacob was really excited. His friend's hair was looking good, but Jacob decided it would be better if he applied a finishing product to define the look. He decided to use a new gloss wax that had arrived that day. He used a large blob of the wax and worked it into the hair. Unfortunately it made his friend's hair look very lank and greasy. He had to offer the service for free – his friend was really disappointed.

- How could Jacob have prevented this from happening?
- Was he right to offer the service for free? Why?

Just checking

1 What is the main purpose of using gel on the hair for styling?
  a To define curl and waves
  b To add volume and style support
  c Provides strong hold to a style and can dry into the hair or be left for a wet look
  d Some hold but mainly adds moisture to the hair for very dry or damaged hair

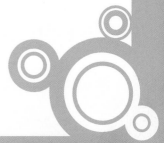

Tools and equipment

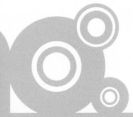

In this topic you will learn about:

- Tools and equipment

Why do you think hairdressers and barbers have so many different combs and brushes?

You will need to be familiar with a range of tools and equipment for styling men's and women's hair. You need to try them all and be trained in their correct use. This is essential under health and safety law. Learn what each one does and the effects you can create when using them.

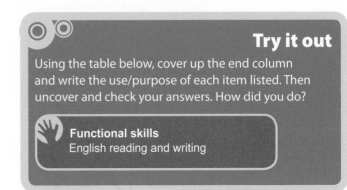

Try it out

Using the table below, cover up the end column and write the use/purpose of each item listed. Then uncover and check your answers. How did you do?

Functional skills
English reading and writing

Tool/equipment	Photo of tool/equipment	Uses/purpose
Combs		Combs are used to detangle the hair or section the hair during styling
Brushes		Round brushes create lift and curl in hair during blow-drying and a paddle brush is used when drying hair straight
Pin tail comb		To take really straight and accurate sections during styling, or for backcombing

Grips and pins	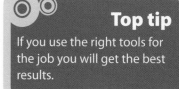	Grips hold the hair in place while styling and pins hold rollers in place while setting
Dryer		For blow-drying hair – can be used with a nozzle for more direct drying
Curling tongs		Can be used to add curls or waves to hair, or spiral curls on longer hair
Straightening irons		Uses high heat to temporarily straighten hair, removes curls and wave (but not permanently)

Just checking

1   What type of comb is best for getting really straight sections?

2   What type of brush should you use to get lift and curl in the hair when blow-drying?

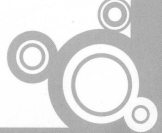

Top tip

If you use the right tools for the job you will get the best results.

Prepare for styling men's and women's hair

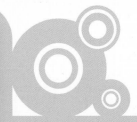

In this topic you will learn about:

- Preparing for the service
- Factors to consider before styling

 Q Why is it important that you have all your tools and equipment ready before your client comes into the salon/barbers for their service?

Before your client arrives, make sure you have all your tools and equipment ready to use. It doesn't give a professional image if you have to keep leaving your client to get things you need.

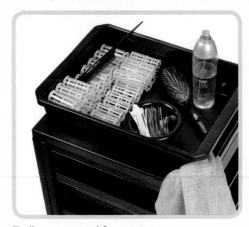

Trolley prepared for setting

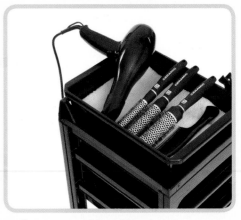

Trolley prepared for blow-drying

When your client arrives, complete a consultation to find out what your client wants and if it's possible to do it.

Look back at the *Anatomy and physiology* unit to remind yourself of the factors that you need to think about before starting the service.

If you are working on a male client, you should also check for **male pattern baldness**.

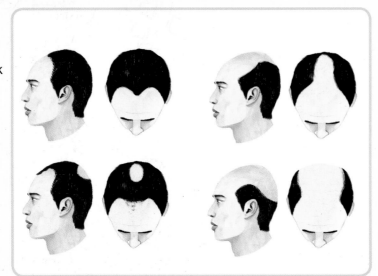

Examples of male pattern baldness

Top tip

If a client has male pattern baldness, think about the way you can style the hair to make it look less noticeable.

Client consultation sheet

Client's name:

Date:

Hair type: curly ☐   wavy ☐   straight ☐

Hair texture: fine ☐   medium ☐   coarse ☐

Hair length: short ☐   medium ☐   long ☐

Face shape:

oval ☐   round ☐   square ☐   long ☐

heart-shaped ☐   pear-shaped ☐   oblong ☐

Hair growth patterns: cowlick ☐   nape whorl ☐

double crown ☐   widow's peak ☐

Adverse hair, skin & scalp conditions:

head lice ☐   eczema ☐   psoriasis ☐

impetigo ☐   dandruff ☐   male pattern baldness ☐

Products used:

Tools & equipment used:

Try it out

Practise your consultation skills on a friend. Your tutor may provide you with a consultation sheet to use while you are learning. Ask your tutor for feedback.

Functional skills
English speaking and listening

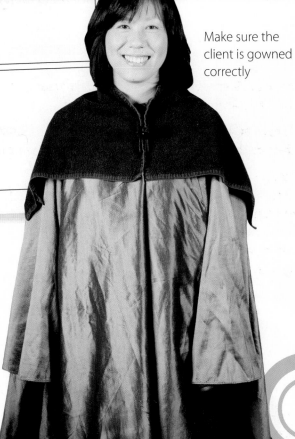

Make sure the client is gowned correctly

Once you have asked the client all the necessary questions, and had a good look at the hair, decide which products, tools and equipment you should use. Most importantly, make sure you understand what the client wants you to do.

Just checking

1 How should your client be prepared for a styling service?

Techniques for styling women's and men's hair (1)

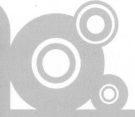

In this topic you will learn about:

- Straightening and smoothing
- Finger drying

Q How many different effects do you think can be achieved by blow-drying?

Straightening and smoothing

This technique can be carried out on both male and female clients. The hair should be blow-dried as straight as possible and straightened to smooth the cuticles, leaving a smooth straight finish.

Blow-drying using a flat brush and straighteners

See page 100 for a blow-drying sequence using round and Denman brushes.

After shampooing and conditioning, towel dry the client's hair and comb through before you begin to section.

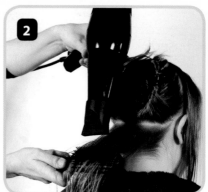

Place the flat brush under the roots of the hair and blow-dry, encouraging root lift and volume. Keep the dry hair from falling onto wet hair.

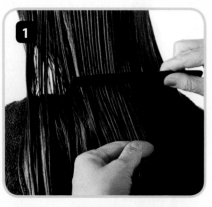

Continue to move through the blow-dry from the nape to the occipital bone. Remember to include the sides of the client's head.

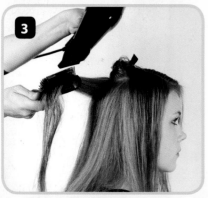

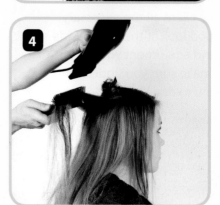

To encourage a smooth and shiny look, direct the dryer down the hair shaft.

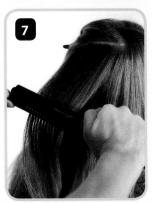
5 Stand parallel to the section you are blow-drying when taking in the sides. Check with the client if they are happy with the style as it develops.

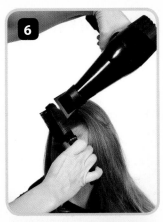

6 Angle the dryer and brush to finish the fringe area.

Top tip

Remember to keep the airflow going from root to point, as this will help to keep the cuticle flat.

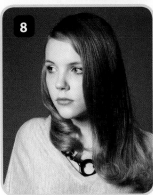
7 Use straighteners and a comb for a polished finish.

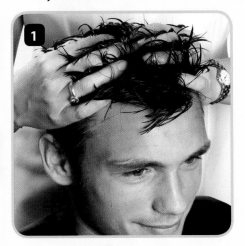
8 The finished look – apply products such as spray or serum to complete the look as required.

Try it out

Using a friend or a mannequin head, blow-dry the hair using a flat brush. Remember to take neat sections and try to control the hair. Ask your tutor to give you feedback and then smooth over the look using straighteners.

Finger drying

Finger drying is usually carried out on short hair, especially men's hair, as they tend to like more a more unstructured look.

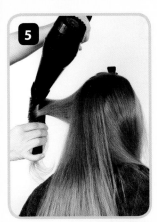
Apply the desired amount of product and distribute evenly through the hair.

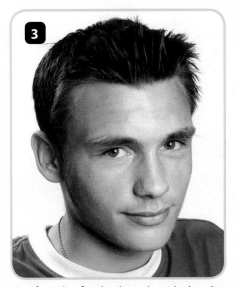
Dry the hair into the desired style, making sure that the hairdryer is at the correct angle. The airflow will then produce the correct amount of root lift.

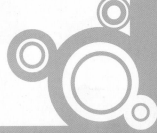
Confirm the finished result with the client.

Just checking

1 Which way should the airflow of the dryer be directed to make sure the final look is smooth and shiny?

Techniques for styling women's and men's hair (2)

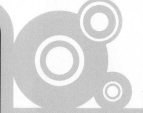

In this topic you will learn about:
- Blow-drying
- Hair up

 For what kind of occasions would a client want a 'hair-up' service?

Blow-drying

There are lots of different looks you can get from blow-drying hair. They range from very curly to straight and smooth and everything in between.

Blow-drying smooth and straight

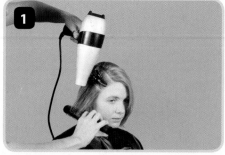

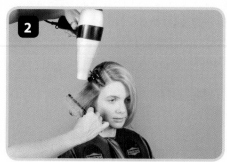

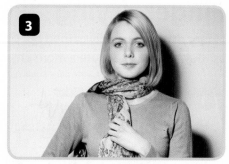

Section the hair into four. Drop a sub-section at the nape and blow-dry under. Then, take each section down and blow-dry up to the crown. Finish with the sides.

Use either a round brush or a Denman brush to smooth the hair at the sides as you continue to work up to the parting.

Allow the hair to cool before you apply finishing products. Check that the balance is right and that your client is happy with the result.

Blow-drying for a curly look

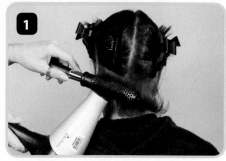

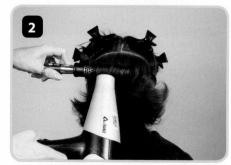

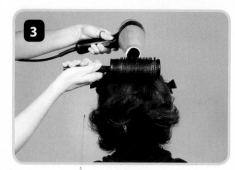

Divide the hair into four and bring down a sub-section of hair in the nape. Blow-dry this section under, in the direction required.

Release one of the main back sections and continue to blow-dry the hair in the desired manner.

At the crown area, blow-dry the hair down, creating body and root lift.

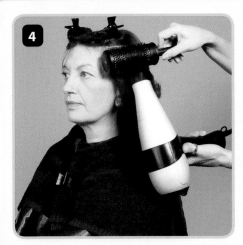

4

Release a section at the side and blow-dry in the desired direction.

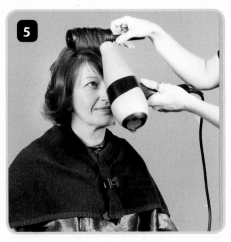

5

From the top sections, continue to join the side sections to achieve a balanced shape.

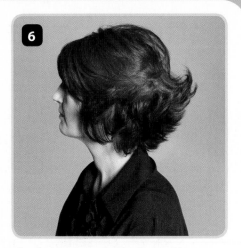

6

The finished result. The hair is blow-dried all over using a slightly cooler heat. Run your fingers through the hair to soften the look. Apply the appropriate finishing products.

Hair up

There are many different ways you can dress long hair into an 'up style'. The key to success is being able to control the hair. You can do this by:

- backcombing the hair
- working in small, controllable sections. If you are trying to deal with too much hair all at once, it can become overwhelming!

One of the easiest hair-up styles is the vertical roll (or French pleat as it's also known).

Top tip

Make sure your sections are straight and the same width as the round brush that you will be using. Each section must be rolled down to sit on its own base.

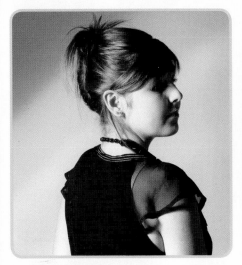

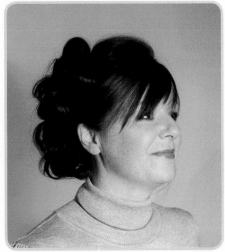

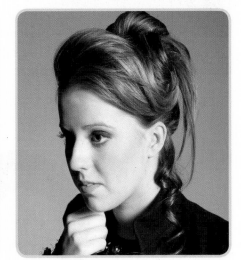

Often the simplest looks are the most stunning. Remember, less is more!

Just checking

1 What should you do to make sure you can control the hair while you're dressing a hair-up style?

Try it out

Ask your tutor to show you other hair-up looks and see how you get on.

Setting the hair

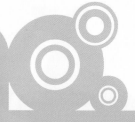

In this topic you will learn about:
- Setting

Q **What kind of effects do you think can be achieved by setting the hair?**

Setting the hair

You can set the hair to achieve curl, lift and volume. This is great for 'big hair' styles. 'Big hair' can be achieved by setting the hair on big rollers that sit on their own base. The hair is then backcombed to support the lift. Other styles involve big bouncy curls or small tight curls. The amount of curl will be decided by the length of the hair and the size of the rollers you use.

How to set the hair

Ask the client how they want the hair to look when it's finished. The rollers should then be placed in the same direction as the hair will fall when it's finished. For example, if the finished look has a parting and side fringe, then the rollers should be placed the same way.

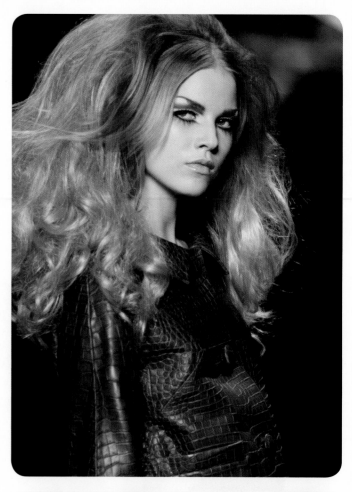

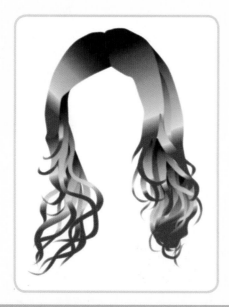

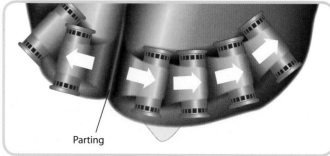

Parting

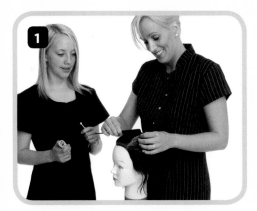

Towel dry and detangle the hair, then comb it in the way you will be styling it.

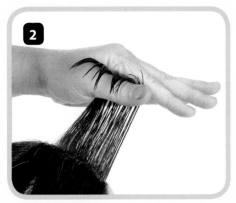

Start at the front hairline. Take a section of hair that is the same size as the roller you are going to use. It is important that your sections are really straight.

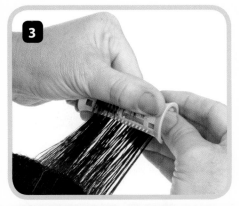

Comb the hair so it is really smooth, and then comb it straight up and slightly forward. Put the roller on the ends of the hair, making sure the ends are smooth and tucked around the roller.

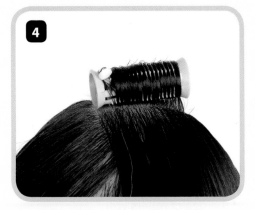

Carefully roll down the roller until it sits on the section you took.

Top tip

Try not to set the rollers in straight lines as this will make it harder for you to hide the roller lines when you come to dress the hair. You should set the hair in either a brickwork pattern or use directional setting.

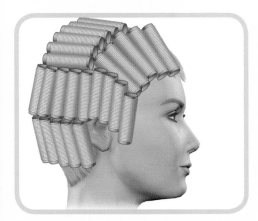

Directional setting

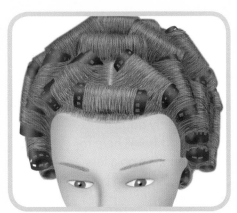

Brickwork technique

Try it out

Using a friend or your mannequin head, have a go at setting the hair. Ask your tutor how you can improve your technique.

Just checking

1 What effects can be achieved by setting the hair?

2 When putting in rollers, what size should each section be?

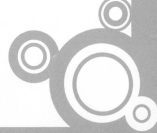

Drying, dressing and pin-curling the hair

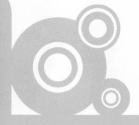

In this topic you will learn about:
- Drying the hair
- Dressing the hair
- Pin curling

When do you think you could use pin curling as a method of curling the hair?

Drying the hair

When you have set the hair, dry it thoroughly under a hood dryer.

Remember to check the time your client is under the dryer. If the hair is over-dried it can be difficult to dress and if it isn't dried properly the set will drop. The length of time will depend on how long the hair is and the size of rollers you used.

When the client's hair is dry, take the client from under the dryer and let the hair cool down. This is done because:
- the hair often feels dry when it's hot but, once it has cooled down, it may still be damp
- it allows the hair to 'set' properly in its new shape.

Dressing the hair

Once the hair is dried, brush it through. Start at the nape and use both a flat brush and a dressing brush. Gently double brush the hair in the direction you have set it. This will help to remove the roller lines. However, if you are working on a less structured or more of a fashion look, you can gently run your fingers through the hair to break up the curls.

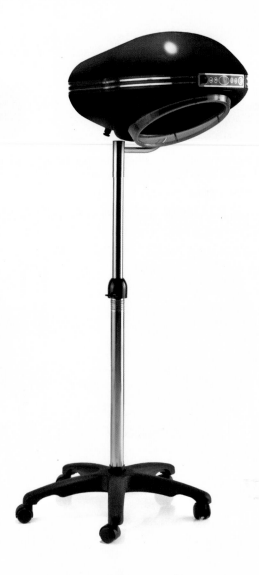

Hood dryer

Pin curling

Pin curling can also be used when setting the hair. Stand up pin curls will give you the same effect as setting.

Top tip

To stop the pin curls from becoming flattened, pop a small piece of cotton wool inside to keep them rounded.

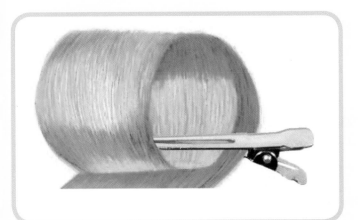

Pin curl

In the salon

David had his first client booked in for a set. He had been practising a lot. He carried out his consultation and prepared the client. He started putting rollers in the hair but each time he put one in, it sprang out. Eventually he called over one of the senior stylists for help. The stylist said that the client had very springy hair and suggested he use pin curls instead. The client was really pleased with the end result. It looked like a set and David had learned how to deal with springy hair.

- Was David right to ask for help?
- What might have happened if he had carried on struggling without asking?

Try it out

Ask your tutor to show you how to do pin curls then try it for yourself on a friend or mannequin's head. Remember to ask your tutor for feedback.

Just checking

1 After the hair had been dried, why should you let it cool down before you start dressing the hair?

2 Why is it important to brush the hair thoroughly after it has been set?

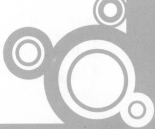

Plaiting and twisting hair

In this unit you will learn about:
- Preparing for hair plaiting and twisting
- Selecting products, tools and equipment for basic plaiting and twisting
- Carrying out plaiting techniques
- Carrying out twisting techniques

Introduction

Plaiting and twisting can add **individuality** to a style. Decoration, such as ribbons or flowers, can be used to give the hair a unique look. On- or off-scalp plaits and twists can be used for everyday looks, but are used more often for special occasion looks.

While learning the different techniques of plaiting and twisting you will become more **dextrous** and creative in your hairdressing work. It will help if you try plaiting and twisting on different types of hair too. You will find it is easier to carry it out on African type hair than Caucasian, which is softer and less **malleable**.

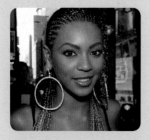
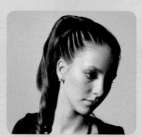
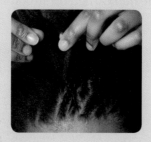

Top tip

The more you practise plaiting and twisting, the easier it will become. Try it on different types of hair, for example, Caucasian and African type. This will help you to develop your skills further.

Key terms

Individuality – something that is different from the norm

Dextrous – skilled with your hands

Malleable – can be shaped easily

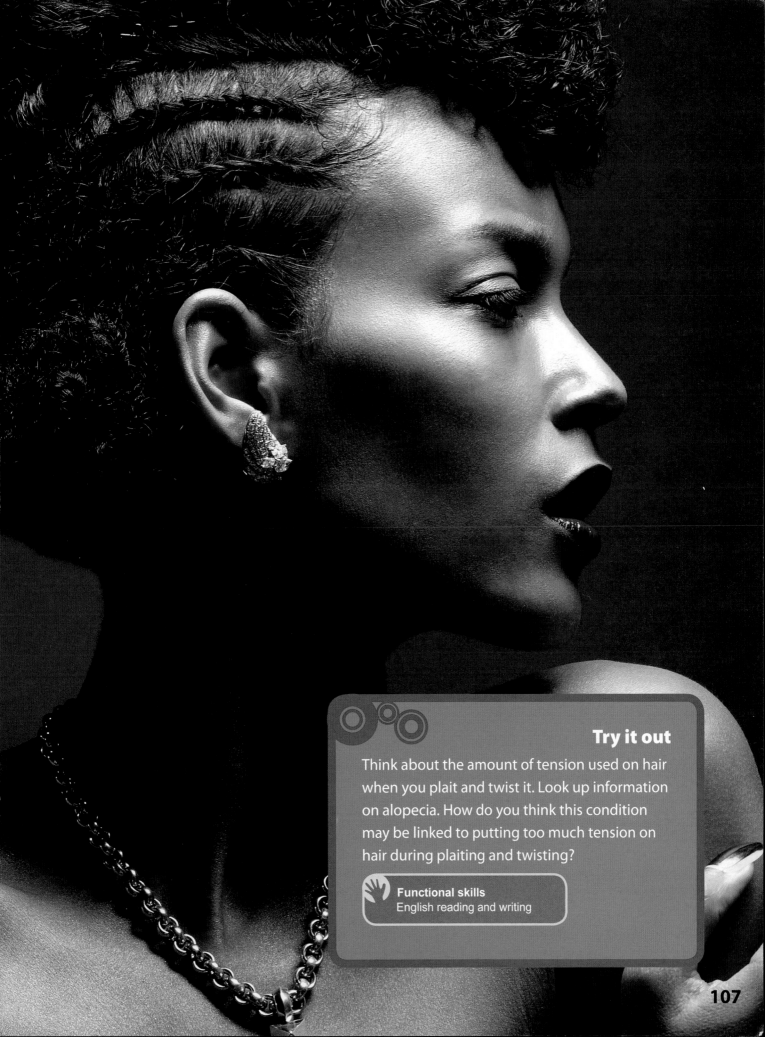

Try it out

Think about the amount of tension used on hair when you plait and twist it. Look up information on alopecia. How do you think this condition may be linked to putting too much tension on hair during plaiting and twisting?

Functional skills
English reading and writing

Prepare for hair plaiting and twisting

In this topic you will learn about:

- Preparing your client and yourself for plaiting and twisting

Q **What does the term PPE mean?**

Protecting the client

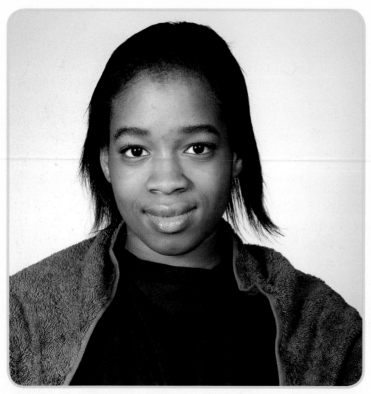

Correct PPE is important to ensure the client's clothes are protected

Use correct **PPE**, such as a clean gown, clean towel, and a plastic cape. This protects the client's clothing from any spillages of product.

Preparing the client's hair

You may need to shampoo the client's hair first, either to clean it or remove product. You must also detangle the hair thoroughly before plaiting and twisting. This is so that you don't hurt the client during the service.

Discuss with the client how they want the finished style to look. While you are doing this, check the scalp and hair for anything you think might cause a problem (for example, cuts, signs of **traction alopecia**, damaged or **porous hair**).

Key terms

PPE – personal protective equipment, used to protect the client or stylist

Traction alopecia – patches of baldness caused by too much tension on the hair

Porous hair – hair that has been weakened or damaged due to cuticle damage

*Use the *Anatomy and physiology* unit to find information on each of these.

Try it out

Think about the things that may affect whether you can plait or twist the hair. Look at the list below. Write down how you think each one may make a difference to the client's plait or twist look:

- Head, face and body shape*
- Lifestyle
- Adverse skin, scalp or hair conditions*
- Hair growth patterns*
- Hair growth cycle*
- Hair length*
- Hair type*

- Texture*
- Elasticity*
- Density*
- Degree of curl*
- Cultural and fashion trends
- Gender*
- Personality
- Occasion

Functional skills
English reading and writing

In the salon

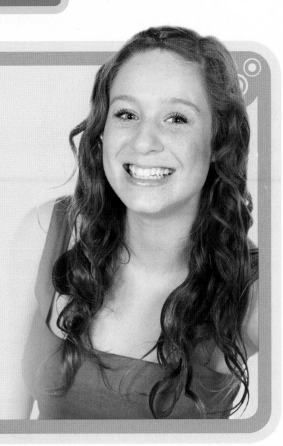

Keeley had a client booked in for a full head of corn row plaits. The client was short in height and Keeley immediately thought that she would have to bend down a lot to do the plaiting work – which could hurt her back. After carrying out the consultation, she explained to the client that she would need to adapt the seating. This was so that she didn't put any strain on her posture or that of the client. She put the chair up to the highest point but this was still too low. After just a few plaits, Keeley's back was starting to ache so she built up the chair with a stack of folded clean towels. This seemed to do the trick, bringing the client to the correct height and easing the strain on her back.

- Was Keeley right to find an alternative way of seating her client or should she have just carried on? How can you make sure your client is comfortable and that your own posture is good?

Just checking

1 Why do you need to check the client's scalp before plaiting and twisting?

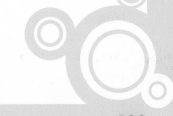

Selecting products, tools and equipment for basic plaiting and twisting

In this topic you will learn about:
- Choosing the right products, tools and equipment when preparing for a plaiting or twisting service
- Ways to improve the look of plaits or twists

Write down different ways you can make plaits or twists look more interesting or exciting.

Products, tools and equipment

If you choose the correct products, tools and equipment, you should find plaiting or twisting hair much easier. Make sure you have everything to hand before you start the service.

Pins

Decorations

Pipe cleaners

Bands

Sectioning clips

Fabrics

Products, tools and equipment

Brushes

Gel

Added hair

Lotions

Oil

Combs

Ribbons and threads

Electrical equipment

Clips

Spray moisturisers

Before you start the plaiting or twisting service, prepare the hair properly. Depending on the look that is wanted, you may have to shampoo, condition and blow-dry or towel dry the hair. Make sure the hair is thoroughly detangled by using either a brush or a wide tooth comb. You may want to blow-dry the hair using the pick or comb attachment, as this will help to detangle the hair and loosen any curls.

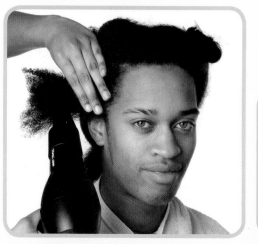

You can use the comb attachment to help loosen the natural curl while blow-drying the hair

Top tip
If you are using electrical equipment, don't forget your responsibilities under the Electricity at Work Regulations.

A pin tail comb should be used to section the hair and to make sure you get even sections.

Products

Using products *during* the styling process will help you to carry out the service. Using them *afterwards* will help to keep the hair in good condition and hold the style in place.

Product	What it does	How it helps
Gel	Helps the styling process by holding the hair in place	It will hold the style in place for longer. It will help to keep stray hairs smooth and tidy.
Oil	Moisturises the hair and scalp Very good on dry, coarse or African type hair	It helps to stop the hair and scalp from drying out and becoming damaged.
Lotions	Moisturises the hair	It adds moisture to the hair.
Moisturisers	Makes the hair look shiny	It adds moisture to the hair and stops it from drying out.
Serum	Smoothes the cuticle	It will help to keep stray hairs smooth and tidy.

Improving the look

You can improve the look of any plait or twist by using ornamentation (decoration) or by adding hair.

Pipe cleaners can be used to add colour to the plait. Because of their flexibility they allow you to bend and twist the whole plait into different shapes.

You can also add hair to your plaits or twists to make the hair look longer. Added hair can introduce other colours to the look too.

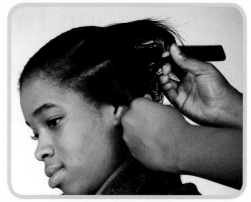

Using a pin tail comb will help you to get straight sections

Fabric

Pipe cleaners

Type of ornamentation

Ribbons

Threads

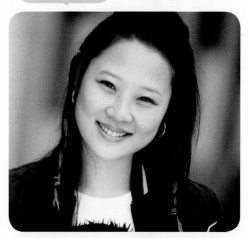

Try it out

Try using different decorations or added hair and see what exciting results you can achieve.

Just checking

1 Why would you use a pin tail comb when carrying out a plaiting service?
   a To hold the hair in place
   b To help you get straight sections
   c To give an exciting look
   d To make the plait stay in longer

Introduction to carrying out plaiting and twisting techniques

In this topic you will learn about:

- On-scalp plaits and off-scalp plaits
- Twisting

Q

Do you know what it feels like to have your hair plaited or twisted? If not, and if your hair is long enough, have it done. You will feel the tension on your head and whether or not it's uncomfortable.

On- and off-scalp plaits

On-scalp plaits are braided to sit snugly to the scalp.

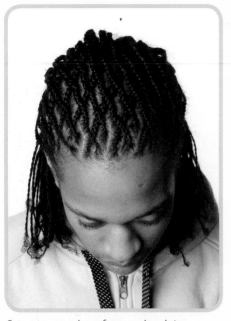 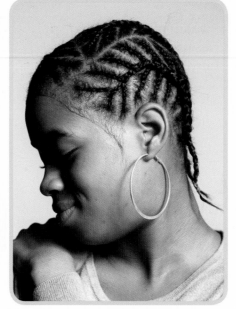 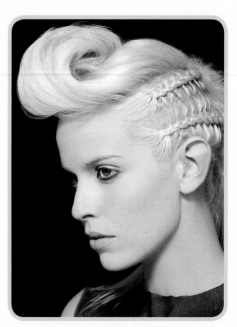

Some examples of on-scalp plaits

Off-scalp plaits are braided by sectioning into two, three or even more sections and plaiting along the length of the hair. The plait is then secured with a band to stop it coming undone.

Try it out

Try out different types of on- and off-scalp plaits on a training head or model. Ask your trainer or assessor to watch and help if you need it.

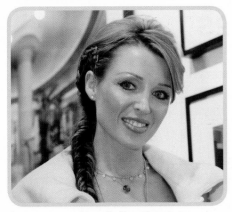
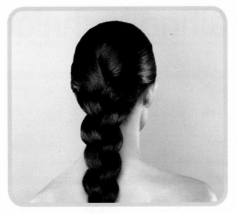
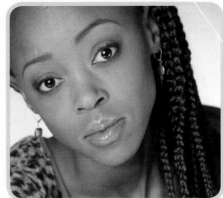

Some examples of off-scalp plaits

Twisting

Twisting is carried out by either twisting the hair in a single stem close to the scalp (flat twist) or off the scalp in a two-strand twist.

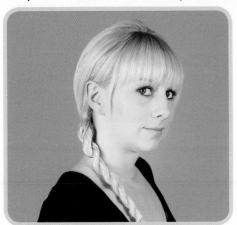
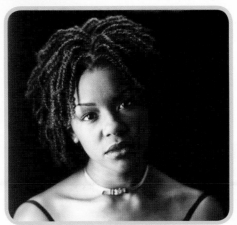

Examples of two-strand twists

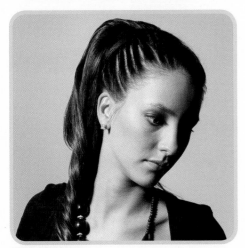

Flat twists

Try it out

Try out different twisting techniques on a training head or model. Again, ask your trainer or assessor to watch and help if you need it.

Top tip

The more you practise all the plaiting and twisting techniques, the easier they become.

Just checking

1 What is the difference between on-scalp and off-scalp plaits?

2 How do twists differ from plaits?

Carrying out plaiting techniques

In this topic you will learn about:

- How to plait hair

Q Why is it important to carry out a thorough consultation before starting a plaiting service?

Before you start your plaiting service, carry out a full consultation with your client. Look back at the *Anatomy and physiology* unit for information on the factors you should be thinking about.

French plait

Top tip

Check the client's hair growth patterns – you will get a much better result if you work with the way the hair falls naturally. You also need to think about the hair's elasticity. If the client wears their hair in plaits most of the time, it could affect the elasticity of the hair. If the elasticity is poor, the hair may break if you apply too much tension.

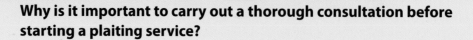
Take a small section from the front hairline and divide into three equal parts

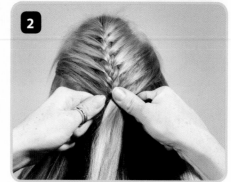
Begin the plait by crossing the hair over each side. Pick up a small section of hair from each side of the head in turn and add to the plait. Continue down the head

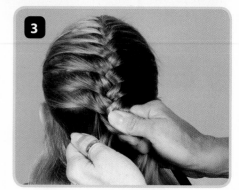
Make sure you keep even tension by holding the hair firmly between the thumb and first finger

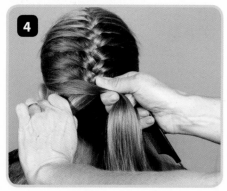
Continue with this routine, adding a small section from each side all the way down the head

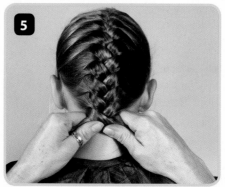
Make sure you maintain even tension all the way to the nape, then continue the plait down to the ends of the hair and secure

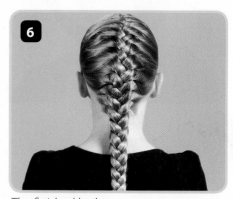
The finished look

Fishtail plait

Try it out

Try out a French plait on a training head or a friend. If you're working on a friend, ask about the tension you have used. Is it comfortable or is their hair being pulled too tight?

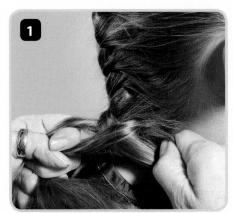

At the end of a French plait – when it reaches the nape – separate the hair into two even sections

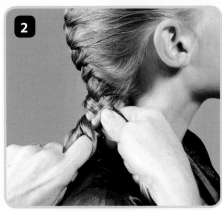

Begin to pass small sections of hair over, keeping even tension

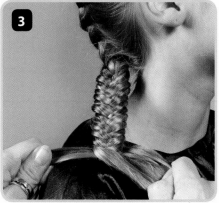

As you work along the length of the hair, keep the sections even and maintain good tension

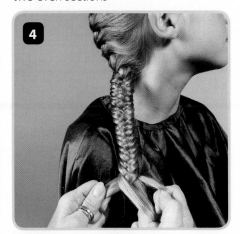

Remember to only take small, even sections along the length of the fishtail plait

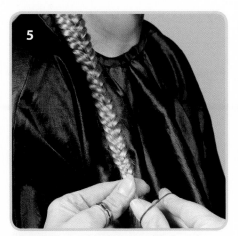

Secure the end with a suitable band

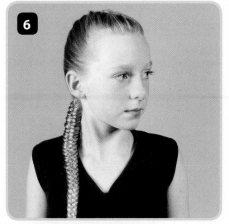

The finished look

Just checking

1 You need to check the client's hair growth patterns before starting the plaiting service because:
   a You should be working with the natural growth patterns
   b You should be working against the natural growth patterns
   c Your tutor has said you should
   d It will help you to decide which products to use.

2 If the hair's elasticity is poor it could lead to:
   a Shiny hair
   b Uneven plaits
   c Breakage
   d Sores on the client's head.

Try it out

Try out a fishtail plait on a friend. Check how your friend feels about your work. Remember you can tell this from what they say, how they say it and their body language.

Carrying out twisting techniques

Q Why should you give your clients aftercare advice?

As with any salon service, talk through what the client wants before starting the twisting service. You should consider all the health and safety factors that may affect the service. Look back at the *Anatomy and physiology* unit for more information.

Twists (like plaits) can be off the scalp or on the scalp. This will depend on the look you are trying to create.

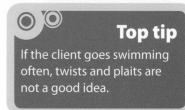

Top tip

If the client goes swimming often, twists and plaits are not a good idea.

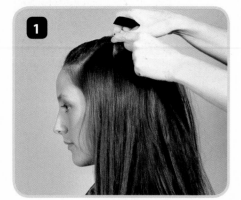

1 Begin by taking a small section of hair from the front hair line towards the crown

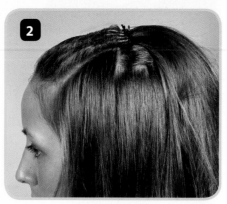

2 Twist each section closely back on itself so it sits snugly against the scalp and secure with Kirby grips

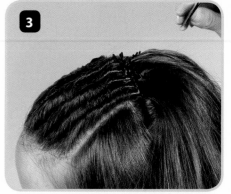

3 Continue this process down from the top of the head to the top of the ear

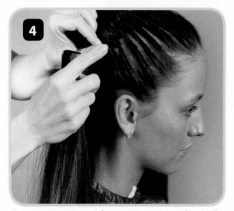

4 As you continue the twists, cross the Kirby grips over each other for a secure hold

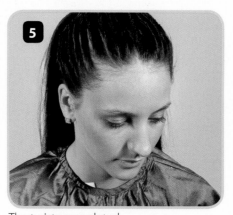

5 The twists completed

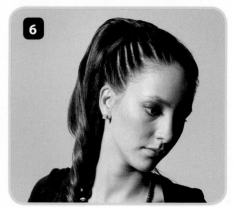

6 You can style the hair that is left out to create a different look; for example, curls or waves

Aftercare advice

It's important that you give your client advice on how to keep their plaits or twists looking good. This will show professionalism and also make sure the client is happy. If you don't give them the right advice, the plaits or twists may not last very long. If the client has had corn row plaits, explain how to care for them. For example, a light oil applied to the scalp will stop it from becoming too dry. An oil based spray applied to the plaits will help keep them looking shiny and stop the hair from becoming dry.

The client needs to avoid anything that rubs or causes friction on the hair because this will leave it looking **matted**.

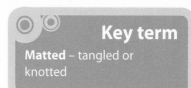

Top tip

At night, the use of a satin or silky pillowcase or headscarf will help to stop the hair from becoming matted. This is because it doesn't cause any friction.

You should also give the client advice on how to remove the plaits or twists. They should start at the ends of the hair and gently unpick the plait using a pin tail comb.

Top tip

Advise the client not to drag out the bands which are used to hold the plaits in the hair.

Once the plaits have been removed, comb through the hair using a wide tooth comb. If the plaits have been in the hair for some time, the client would benefit from a deep conditioning treatment.

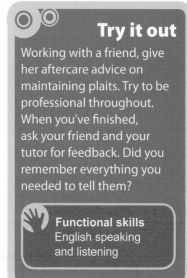

Try it out

Working with a friend, give her aftercare advice on maintaining plaits. Try to be professional throughout. When you've finished, ask your friend and your tutor for feedback. Did you remember everything you needed to tell them?

Functional skills
English speaking and listening

Just checking

1. When removing scalp plaits, advise the client to start at the:
   a   Roots
   b   Points
   c   Front
   d   Back.

2. So that the plaits or twists last as long as possible, when the client goes to bed you should suggest that they use:
   a   A woolly hat
   b   A silk scarf
   c   A baseball cap
   d   A beanie hat.

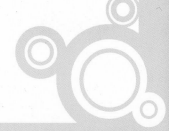

The art of dressing hair

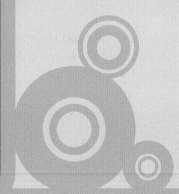

In this unit you will learn about:

- Consulting with the client and evaluating the hair
- Styling products, tools and equipment
- Preparation for dressing hair
- Long hair looks
- Styling and dressing hair including blow-drying, finger drying, using a diffuser, brickwork and directional setting, pin curling, finger waving, using tongs, heated rollers and straighteners
- Structural hair changes and the effects of humidity
- Aftercare

Introduction

An important part of all hair services is the styling to finish off the client's hair. Whatever service they have had, whether it is colouring, cutting or perming, they will always need their hair finishing off professionally. This will involve using techniques such as blow-drying, setting, finger drying, straightening and dressing long hair. Each of these is covered in more detail within the unit. You will also need to know how styling affects the hair structure and the different products available for use to add **volume**, straighten or fight the **effects of humidity**.

Top tip

Good product knowledge will mean you always use the right product to hold the style in place for longer.

Key terms

Volume – putting root lift and movement into the hair

Effects of humidity – how moisture in the air affects the style holding in place

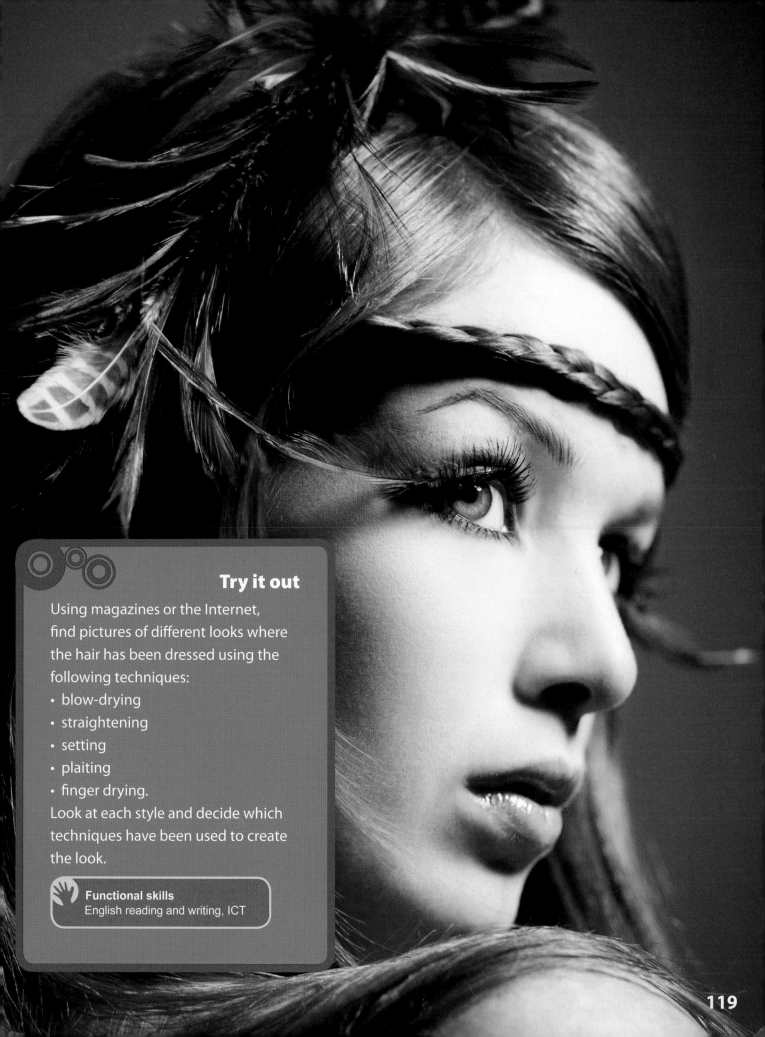

Try it out

Using magazines or the Internet, find pictures of different looks where the hair has been dressed using the following techniques:

- blow-drying
- straightening
- setting
- plaiting
- finger drying.

Look at each style and decide which techniques have been used to create the look.

Functional skills
English reading and writing, ICT

Consult with client and evaluate the hair

In this topic you will learn about:
- Asking questions to find out what the client wants
- Using visual aids to help with your consultation
- Finding out about fashion trends

 List the things you need to find out about a client's hair before you start styling and dressing their hair.

You must carry out a thorough consultation with your client before starting a style and dress service. This is to make sure you understand what the client wants from the service. It will also help you to decide whether it's possible to achieve the look they want.

Asking questions

The best way to find out what the client wants is to ask questions. Ask open questions. If you do, you will be given fuller answers.

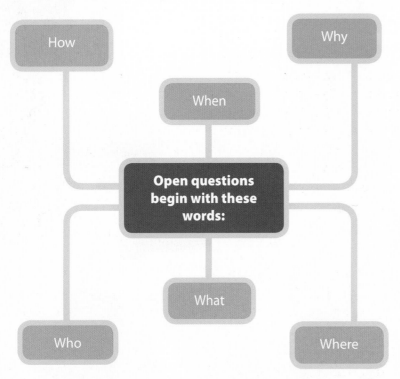

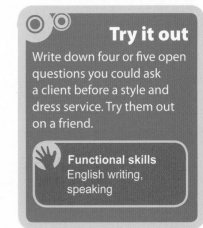

Try it out

Write down four or five open questions you could ask a client before a style and dress service. Try them out on a friend.

Functional skills
English writing, speaking

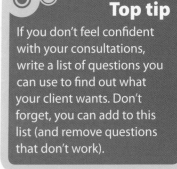

Top tip

If you don't feel confident with your consultations, write a list of questions you can use to find out what your client wants. Don't forget, you can add to this list (and remove questions that don't work).

Closed questions only need a 'yes' or 'no' response. For example, 'Do you want your hair blow-dried today?' is a closed question.

Using visual aids

Clients don't always find it easy to explain what they want, so using visual aids such as a style book or magazine can make it much easier for them and you.

Fashion trends

Make sure you are up to date with what is fashionable. This is so you can identify a new style, product or styling technique that your client asks for. You can do this by:

- going to training sessions
- watching TV (especially the fashion/lifestyle channels)
- reading magazines, especially those related to hairstyles, styling and celebrities
- using the Internet.

By doing this, the client will feel more confident that you can do their hair.

Refer to the *Anatomy and physiology* unit for information on factors that you should consider during consultation.

Remember, your body language should be positive when you're carrying out any service.

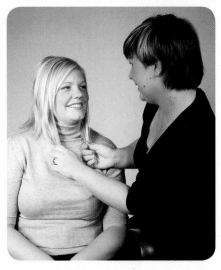

Positive body language will make the client feel comfortable

Key term

Walk-in client – a client who does not have an appointment

In the salon

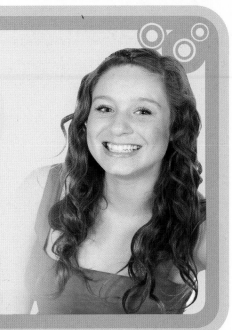

Keeley was asked to carry out a blow-dry service on a **walk-in client**. She had a quick chat with the client then shampooed her hair. She started to blow-dry the client's hair and it was looking good. However, the expression on the client's face showed she was really unimpressed. Keeley thought the client might be having a bad day. She continued the service and smiled all the way through so she looked professional. When she had finished, she was really pleased with what she had done. She asked the client if she liked it and the client replied that it was OK, but not what she wanted. However, it would have to do, as she had an appointment in 15 minutes. Keeley was very upset.

- What did Keeley do wrong? If you were the client, what would you have done? What should Keeley do in the future to make sure that it never happens again?

Just checking

1 When you want to find out information from a client, you should use:
   a Closed questions   b Ajar questions
   c Open questions   d Leading questions.

2 You can find out about current fashion trends by:
   a Attending school   b Researching on the Internet
   c Watching cartoons on TV d Listening to the radio.

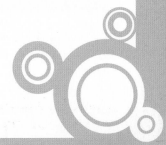

Styling products

In this topic you will learn about:

- Styling products used when dressing hair

You will probably have used a variety of different styling products. Write a list of your favourites and another list of new products that you would like to try on clients.

Most clients are happy for you to try something new in their hair. It gives them a chance to check if they like the product before they buy it – but remember to always ask first.

Styling products used when dressing hair

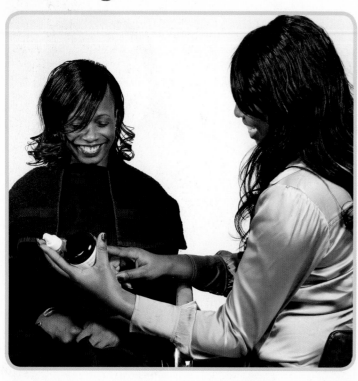

Let clients try your styling products – it may encourage them to buy

Top tip

Ask the wholesalers or company reps for free samples so you can try the products first, either on your own hair or on a willing client. You can then decide if the styling products will do what they say.

Try it out

Look at the product range in the salon and read the manufacturers' instructions. Make notes on all the benefits that the products offer. Don't forget to tell clients about them.

Functional skills
English reading and writing

The products we use when styling hair fall into two types: styling products and finishing products. Styling products are used to make the hair easier to work with while styling. They also help to fight humidity and hold the style in place. Finishing products hold the style in place and add shine or gloss to the hair.

The table below offers you plenty of information on styling products.

Product	Uses	Comments
Lotions	Used before blow-drying or setting on wet hair. Available in light to firm hold	Some contain chemicals that protect the hair from heat
Mousse	Spread evenly through wet hair. Available in light to firm hold. Adds volume and body to the hair	May contain UV filters and protects the hair from humidity
Activator	Any styling product that has an active ingredient; for example, to fight humidity or activate natural curl	Fights the effects of humidity, defines curl, adds moisture or shine
Gel	Apply to wet hair and spread evenly. Gives a firm hold, especially good when finger waving	Ideal for short, textured styles and for moulding the hair into place
Moisturiser	Apply to wet hair before styling. Makes hair soft and shiny and more manageable	Useful on dry or damaged hair to add shine and make the hair appear healthier
Sprays	Used to hold a style in place and as long as it is not over applied can be brushed out easily	Supplied in different strengths depending on how much hold you require; for example, light, firm, ultra
Wax	Apply after drying to add texture or movement to the hair, or to define curl	Take care not to overload the hair or you will have to shampoo out and start again
Serum	Used on dry or brittle hair to help restore moisture and add shine. Also adds some definition to a style	Do not apply on root area as may make the hair feel greasy. On fine hair it will weigh down the hair and make styling difficult
Dressing cream	Has a light hold and is used either lightly to smooth down stray hairs after styling or heavily to create a slicked down look	Can leave the hair sticky to touch
Oils	For use on very course, dry hair only. Will add moisture and shine but has no hold	Can also be used after cutting patterns into the hair to add definition

Just checking

1 What are the two main types of products available for dressing hair?
2 What is likely to happen if serum is applied to finer hair?

Top tip

All of the styling products you use are likely to be flammable or toxic. Take care not to use them near a naked flame or heat, for example, hot irons. Do not leave them where they can be reached by young visitors. Be aware of COSHH regulations for the products you use.

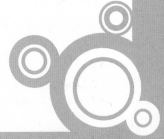

Styling tools and equipment

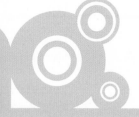

In this topic you will learn about:
- Tools, equipment and accessories used when dressing hair

Write a list of the tools and equipment you might use when dressing hair. Compare your list with the table below. Have you missed any or have you thought of others that are not listed here?

There are many different tools, equipment and accessories that you can use while styling your clients' hair. Keep up to date with new trends and try these out in training sessions so you will always be able to offer the latest looks.

Top tip
Carry out proper training in using any new tools or equipment before using them on your clients. This follows health and safety regulations.

Tools and equipment

Tools and equipment		Correct use	Routine maintenance
Hand-held dryer with nozzle		This is used to blow-dry hair. Take care not to direct onto the scalp as this will burn the client. The nozzle allows more directed drying.	Unplug the dryer and wipe over with an alcohol-based wipe. Clean the vent at the back and then put it back on.
Hood dryer		Used to dry hair that has been set. Don't leave too high or you will burn the client.	Unplug the dryer and wipe over with an alcohol-based wipe. Dust the hood over each day.
Diffuser		Attach to a hand-held dryer in place of nozzle to dry curly hair without too much disturbance.	Remove from the dryer and wipe over with an alcohol-based wipe.
Flat brushes		Used to blow-dry hair straight (good for longer hair) or for dressing out following setting.	Pull out any hair then wash and dry and place in a UV cabinet.
Round brushes		Used when blow-drying to add curl and volume. Take care to use the right size or it may tangle in the hair.	Pull out any hair then wash and dry and place in a UV cabinet.

Rollers secured with pins		Used during setting to add curl, wave or volume. Take care on long hair not to tangle in the hair.	Pull out any hair then wash and dry and place in a UV cabinet.
Pin curl clips		Used when curling shorter styles or finger waving. Take care not to touch the skin as they may burn during drying.	Pull out any hair then wash and dry and place in a UV cabinet.
Straighteners		Used to smooth out and straighten hair after blow-drying. Take care not to burn the hair or skin due to very high temperature.	Unplug them and wipe over with an alcohol-based wipe.
Curling tongs		Used to create curls, wave or volume in hair that has been dried. Take care not to burn the hair or skin due to very high temperature.	Unplug them and wipe over with an alcohol-based wipe.
Heated rollers		Used on dry hair only to create curls, wave or volume. Take care when placing in the hair as they can become quite hot.	Remove any hair from the rollers, clean them carefully and place in a UV cabinet.

Accessories

There are lots of accessories that you can use in your clients' hair. It's a good idea to practise and learn how to use the basic accessories such as feathers, ribbons and flowers.

Most accessories will need a secure base to attach to and you may have to backcomb a mesh of hair to create this base.

You should also tell clients how to remove accessories carefully at home so that they don't damage or tear their hair. For example, clips or grips should be taken out by pushing out from the tips, and knots in ribbons should be untied gently to avoid too much dragging on the hair.

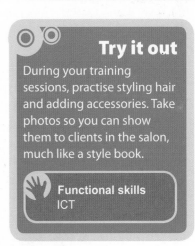

Try it out

During your training sessions, practise styling hair and adding accessories. Take photos so you can show them to clients in the salon, much like a style book.

Functional skills
ICT

Just checking

1 State the correct way to clean a hand-held dryer.

2 How should you check that hair accessories are secure in a client's hair?

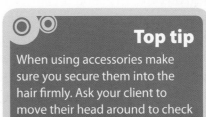

Top tip

When using accessories make sure you secure them into the hair firmly. Ask your client to move their head around to check they are not loose before leaving the salon.

Preparation for dressing hair

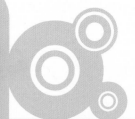

In this topic you will learn about:

- Setting up the work area
- Client preparation
- Positioning of self and client

Do you know how to set up a trolley for a dressing hair service? List the equipment needed for both setting and blow-drying.

Setting up the work area

Once you have carried out a thorough consultation, you must prepare your work area and the client for the service. If you are not fully prepared, you will present an unprofessional image to the client.

In the salon

Navin was taking a lunch break in the salon. A client called in and asked if he could put up her hair into a French pleat. Navin was halfway through his sandwich but said 'yes' as the service wouldn't take long and he didn't have any other clients.

He showed the client to the station and gowned her up. Then he popped in the back to quickly finish his sandwich. When he returned the client wasn't looking too happy and asked him to put her pleat in as quickly as possible. Just then the phone rang. Navin answered it because he was the only person in the salon at that time. When he came back, the client was stony faced. Navin tried to ignore this and went to gather all the tools and equipment he needed. The client now wanted to know how much longer it would take. Navin said it would be about 20 minutes. At this, the client threw off her gown and stormed out saying she couldn't wait that long because she had a job interview and would be late.

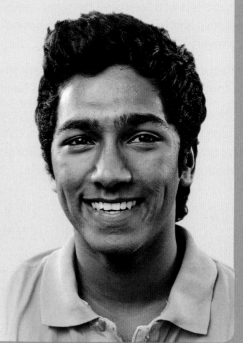

- Should Navin have accepted the client during his lunch break? Could he have been clearer about how long the service would take, including preparation time? What could happen if the client told her friends about how unhappy she was with the service at the salon?

See page 96 for examples of a trolley set up for setting and for blow-drying.

Client preparation/correct PPE

As a minimum, the correct PPE to use when dressing hair is a gown and towel for the client. This is to prevent any spillages onto the client's clothing, which may cause damage. It is likely that you will need an apron and gloves, depending on what products you are using, for example, oils.

Correct positioning of self and client

It is very important to keep good **posture** in the salon to prevent any long-term injury or **fatigue**. You should always work with a good **weight distribution** over both legs and not over stretch yourself over your client. You can do this by positioning the client at the correct working height for you.

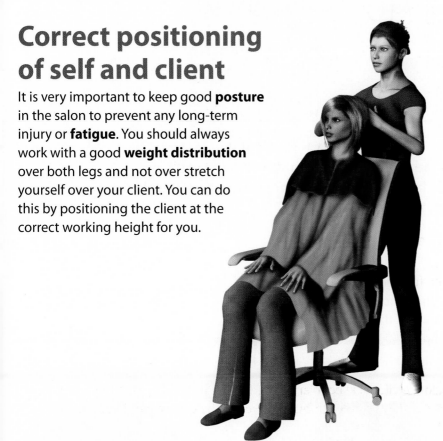

When you are working in the salon, ask someone to check your posture. Is it correct? If not, why not? Think about your posture while you are working and try to improve it.

Just checking

1 What items might you find on a trolley ready for setting?
   a Rollers
   b Perm rods
   c Heated rollers
   d Pin curl clips

2 What are the effects of incorrect posture on you as a stylist?
   a Increased energy
   b Fatigue
   c Aches and pains
   d Dermatitis

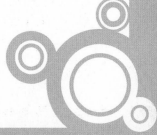

Long hair looks – vertical roll and scalp plait

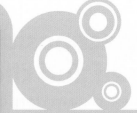

In this topic you will learn about:

- How to carry out a vertical roll (French pleat)
- How to carry out a scalp plait

Q **Have you already tried putting up long hair? Perhaps you have long hair yourself or friends to practise on? The more you work on long hair, the easier it becomes!**

Vertical roll (or French pleat)

The hair is swept up and rolled up the back of the head, vertically. The ends can be tucked in or left out. If left out, you can either curl them or straighten and spike out. Have a look at these step-by-step photos.

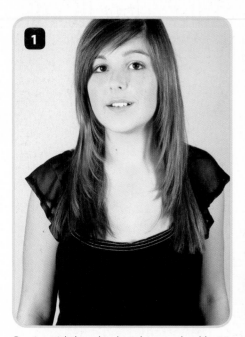
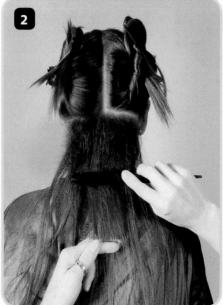
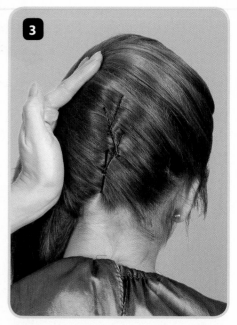

Begin with brushed and unwashed hair

Section the hair and add a little back brushing or back combing to give a good base for the French pleat

Lightly brush over the top section and begin by lifting the hair from the nape and pinning off centre

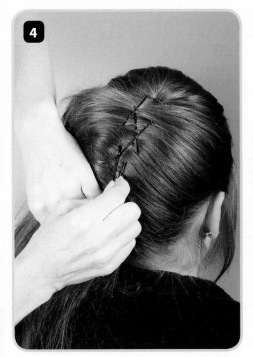

4

Continue to secure the hair up the back of the head, using Kirby grips – these can be crossed over each other for a firmer grip

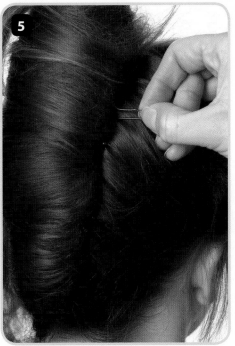

5

Wrap the hair over and tuck under to give a roll up the back of the head – secure using both Kirby grips and fine hair pins

Try it out

On a training head, carry out different types of plaits. Ask your tutor or salon trainer to check your work to let you know how you have done.

Scalp plait

The hair is plaited tight to the head using all of the hair, so it sits close to the scalp. It can be either a full head or partial head. The step-by-step photos on page 114 in *Plaiting and twisting hair* feature a French plait that is a single inverted plait, using all of the client's hair.

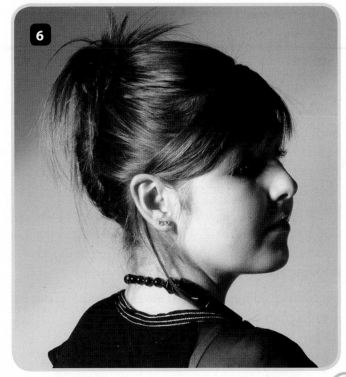

6

The finished look

Just checking

1 A French plait is described as:
  a A plait that sits snugly to the scalp
  b A plait that is a single inverted plait using all the hair
  c A roll up the back of the head
  d A short plait at the front hairline.

2 A vertical roll is described as:
  a A plait that sits snugly to the head
  b A two-stem plait down the hair length
  c A roll up that is secured up the back of the head
  d The use of added hair to build up the length of the hair.

Long hair looks – twists, backcombing and back brushing

In this topic you will learn about:

- How to carry out twists
- Backcombing and back brushing

 Have you ever had your hair backcombed or back brushed? If so, how easy was it to brush or comb out afterwards?

Twists

These can be used on a full head or partial head depending on the style required. The hair is sectioned into narrow straight channels and then swept up and twisted, (like a very small vertical roll). The hair is then secured with grips so the twist doesn't come undone. They sit very close to the scalp in the same way that scalp plaits do.

See page 116 in *Plaiting and twisting hair* for step-by-step photos of twisting.

Backcombing and back brushing

Both backcombing and back brushing can be a little worrying to carry out at first. It's hard to know much pressure to apply and if it will hurt the client. However, most clients that have this service have had it done before and will be used to the tension you need to use on the hair.

The amount of backcombing and back brushing you do depends on the look you are trying to create. Wherever you place it in the hair, it will add volume, so you need to think about the shape you are trying to create and backcomb or back brush to underpin the volume you need.

For both techniques it should always be brushed out thoroughly before shampooing to avoid tangling the hair.

 Top tip

Check with your client that you're not hurting them so you know how much tension it is safe to use.

 Try it out

Using a friend or training head, have a go at twisting the hair. Remember to keep your tension even or the twists won't look neat. When you have finished, ask your friend and/or your tutor for feedback.

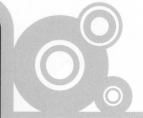

Backcombing

Backcombing is carried out to support the root area of the hair when creating lift and volume. It can also be used to create a pad of hair to attach accessories to.

- Section off the hair.
- Comb a **mesh of hair** up from the scalp. Hold the ends firmly in one hand and use a fine tooth comb (for example, a pin tail comb) to comb the hair from mid-lengths to roots.
- Some of the hair will be pushed down towards the root area, creating a supporting pad of hair at the roots.
- The hair can then be styled over this section to create the volume and lift needed.
- Backcombing along the whole length of the hair may be carried out if the hair is very fine or too soft to work with. This will create even more volume by raising the cuticles so the surface of the hair is roughened.

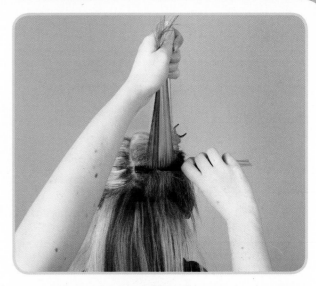

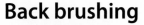

Key term

Mesh of hair – a section of hair taken at the roots

Back brushing

Back brushing is carried out in the same way as backcombing but you use a small, flat, bristle brush instead of a comb. It is more suitable for longer hair as it gives a softer effect. It can be carried out on the top or underneath sections, depending on the look you are trying to achieve.

Show your clients how to remove the backcombing or back brushing without damaging the hair. Do this by brushing from the points to the roots, working gently up the hair.

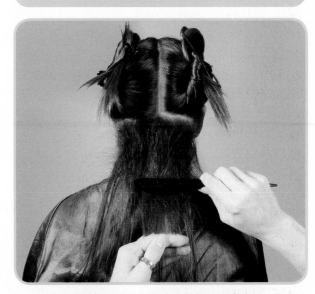

Just checking

1 Why is backcombing/back brushing carried out?
   - a To smooth the hair
   - b To add volume
   - c To make sure the hair is properly dry
   - d To create a pad of hair to secure accessories to

2 What part of the hair structure is affected during back combing?

3 What type of brush should be used during back brushing?
   - a Flat brush
   - b Large, round circular brush
   - c Small, Denman brush
   - d Flat, bristle brush

Top tip

Use good-quality combs and brushes to avoid tearing or damaging the hair. You should also warn your client that using these techniques too often may damage the hair.

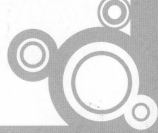

The art of dressing hair   **131**

Blow-drying

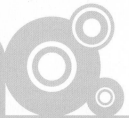

In this topic you will learn about:
- Blow-drying hair

Q **What effects can you achieve from a blow-dry service?**

Blow-drying

You can blow-dry the hair smooth and straight or blow-dry to achieve curls.

Divide the hair into neat, straight sections. This will make it easier to blow-dry and you will get a better result.

Always direct the airflow from root to point, following the way the cuticle lies. This will help the cuticles to lie flat and makes the hair look shiny and healthy. You should also consider the temperature and speed setting of the dryer.

Always blow-dry the hair in the direction it will fall when the style is finished as this will make it:
- easier to dress at the end
- last longer for the client
- easier for the client to manage.

The photos below show blow-drying using round and Denman brushes (see pages 98–99 for a blow-drying sequence using a flat brush and straighteners).

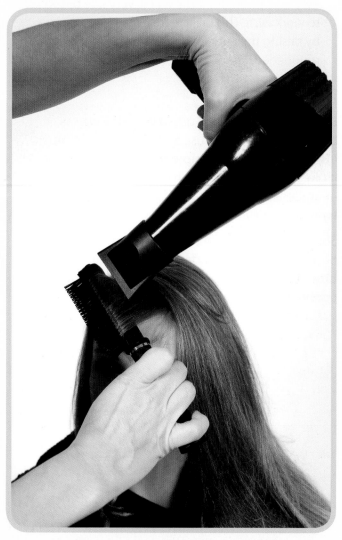

Drying from root to point

Top tip

While you are learning, keep the dryer on the medium settings. This will stop you over-drying the hair and damaging the cuticles. Hair that has been over-dried looks dry and brittle and tends to become flyaway and difficult to manage. By using the medium speed setting, you will have more control of the hair. Remember to keep your dryer moving so you don't burn the client's scalp!

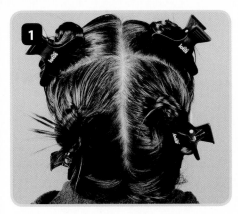

1

Section the shampooed hair into four sections

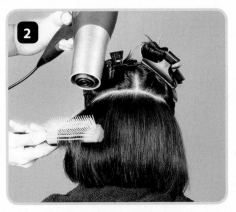

2

Begin the blow dry in the nape area and work up the head, taking sections of about 1–2cm. Use a denman brush to keep the hair smooth

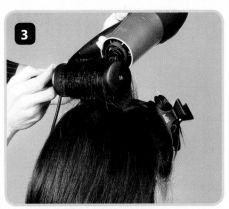

3

As you continue up the head, change to a large round brush at the crown area to add some volume

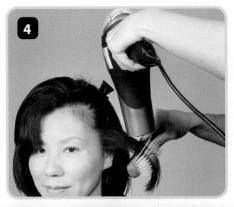

4

Introduce the hair at the sides and work up from the ear to the top of the head – use a denman brush and take sections of 1–2cm

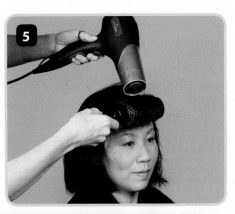

5

Blow-dry the fringe last, using a large round brush to add volume

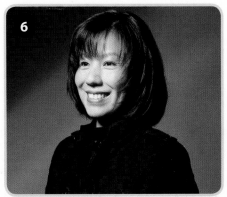

6

The finished look

When you are blow-drying hair, it is important to use the correct tension. You also need to use the correct size of section to suit the hair and the styling service. This makes sure that:

- the heat can go through the section of hair making sure the hair is dried all the way through
- the section of hair suits the length and width of the brush you are using
- you get an even result.

See page 100 in *Styling women's and men's hair* for a step-by-step sequence for blow-drying layered hair.

Just checking

1 When blow-drying, which way should you direct the airflow?

2 Why must you use the correct-size section for both the hair and styling service?

Try it out

You need to be able to work with both hands when you are blow-drying. By doing this, you will get less tired and keep a better posture. Try holding the dryer in your left hand and the brush in your right hand while blow-drying a few sections of hair. Now swap over and blow-dry a few more sections. Keep practising until it feels natural.

Top tip

If you are blow-drying the hair into curls using a small, circular brush, make sure you let the hair cool before brushing it through. This will allow the hair to set into the curl.

Styling and dressing hair (1)

In this topic you will learn about:

- Finger drying
- Drying hair with a diffuser
- Finger waving

Q Have you ever dried curly hair before? Can you think why we use a diffuser attachment to blow-dry curly hair?

Using a diffuser

Use a diffuser to dry permed or naturally curly hair to encourage it to curl without looking frizzy. The hair should be separated into manageable sections. Then scrunch the hair with your hand and place it in the diffuser. The diffuser then sits on the scalp while you move it around in small circles. This allows the heat to circulate. Remember to remove the diffuser at regular intervals and scrunch the hair to see how it's looking. If necessary, put the hair back into the diffuser until it feels almost dry.

Top tip

Scrunch mousse into the hair before drying it with a diffuser. The correct finishing products will give an amazing look to the hair.

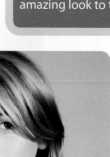
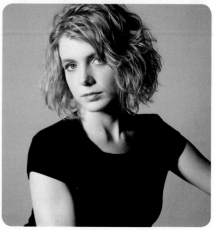

Using a diffuser – before and after

Finger drying

Finger drying is best done on short hair that has some **natural movement**.

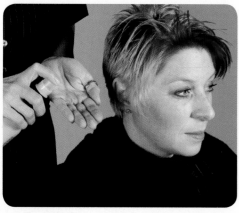

Apply a small amount of styling product to your hands and spread through the hair

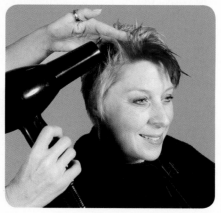

Use your fingers to mould the hair and lift the roots

Key terms

Natural movement – hair that is not straight
Textured – natural or non-structured

When you have dried all the hair, run your fingers through it to give it a **textured** look. You can also use a vent brush to achieve a textured look and then use some wax to finish off.

Finger waving

Finger waving gives flat waves in the hair with no root lift. The hair is moulded into 'S' shapes using your fingers and a straight comb. The hair should be kept wet throughout the styling process to make it easier to get good results.

When doing a finger waved style, use strong styling products to hold the hair in place.

Try it out

Practise finger waving on a head block for both wet hair using gel and dry hair after wet setting and brushing out. Ask your tutor for advice on how you are doing.

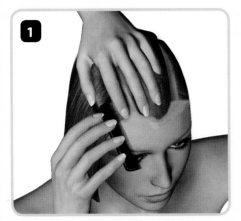

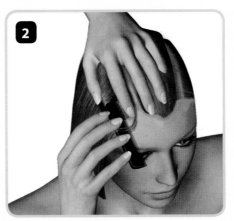

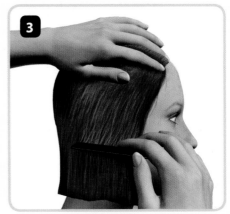

The hair is moulded into 'S' shaped waves using the fingers and a straight comb. To form the first crest, comb the hair downwards and then push the hair away to the left. Pinch the hair between your index and middle fingers to hold the crest in place.

Hold the wave that you've just made, then comb the hair downwards and push it away to the right. Pinch the new crest between your middle and index fingers.

Repeat as before, working around the head until all the hair has been completed.

Just checking

1 What sort of hair would you use a diffuser to dry?

2 What kind of results can you achieve from finger drying the hair?
   a Natural or non-structured
   b Corkscrew curls
   c Augmented waves
   d Highlighted curls

3 Finger waving will produce:
   a Tight curls
   b Loose curls
   c Flat waves with no root lift
   d Flat waves with root lift.

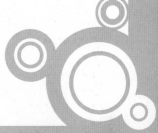

Styling and dressing hair (2)

In this topic you will learn about:
- Setting the hair using brickwork and directional setting
- Pin curling

Look at a selection of photos of celebrities with curly hair. Decide if you think you could achieve a similar look using pin curls?

Setting the hair

Setting the hair gives **root lift**, **curl and volume**.

You can set the hair using rollers with pins, Velcro rollers or heated rollers with pins. Each type of roller comes in different sizes. The length of the client's hair, and how curly the client wants it, will help you to decide what size roller to use. Big rollers will give a soft curl and are better to use on long hair. Small rollers will give a smaller, tighter curl on short hair.

See page 103 in *Styling women's and men's hair* for step-by-step directions on how to place rollers.

Don't set the hair in straight lines, like a ladder, as this can be difficult to dress. Instead you need to use directional and brickwork setting.

Brickwork setting ensures there are no roller lines showing when you dress out the set. It looks like the pattern that is made when bricks are laid. (See page 103.)

Directional setting is done when a client wants their hair to be styled in a certain direction. For example, if the client wants a fringe, place the rollers in the way the style will be dressed when it's finished. (See page 103.)

When you have finished the set, place a net over the rollers before the client goes under the dryer. How long the client spends under the dryer will depend on the length and density of their hair and the size of the rollers.

Key terms
Root lift – where the hair is bouncy at the roots
Curl and volume – where the hair looks fuller, 'big hair'

Top tip
The hair will feel hot when it first comes out of the dryer and you may think it's dry. Check a few rollers around the crown area to make absolutely sure. If the hair is not fully dry, the style will flop.

Try it out
Use a training head or model to set the hair using brickwork or directional setting. Ask your tutor to demonstrate dressing the set.

In the salon

Keeley's friend was going out and wanted big bouncy curls. Keeley needed a model so she offered to set her hair. She was methodical throughout the setting process. All the rollers were sitting on their own bases and it looked really good when she put her friend under the dryer. The setting had taken a bit longer than she thought so after 20 minutes she took her friend out from under the dryer. She checked a roller on the crown to make sure it was properly dry. It felt OK so she took out all the rollers and started to gently brush it through. But the big bouncy curls dropped into limp waves. Keeley's boss felt the hair. He said it wasn't dry, so all that time and effort had been wasted. Her friend was very upset as she didn't have time for Keeley to sort things out.

- What did Keeley do wrong? How would you feel if you were Keeley's friend?

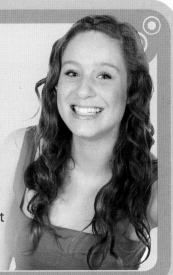

Pin curling

There are different types of pin curls and they can be used to achieve different effects.

Type of pin curl		Effects created
Stand up barrel curl	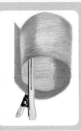	Stand up barrel curls create lift and volume which can produce soft waves or curls. They can be used instead of setting rollers.
Flat barrel curl	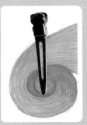	Flat barrel curls sit flat on the head with an open middle. They produce a curl that is even from root to point. This will give flat movement.
Clockspring curl	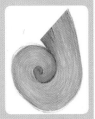	Clockspring curls also sit flat on the head and have a closed centre. They produce a tight curl on the ends with looser curl at the roots. They are usually used in the nape on soft hair.

Just checking

1. Which pin curl would you use to achieve tight curls in the nape?
2. Why do we leave the hair to cool before brushing out curls or waves?

Styling and dressing hair (3)

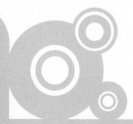

In this topic you will learn about:

- Styling hair using tongs, heated rollers and straighteners
- Checking the balance

 Why should you use a back mirror when you've finished styling the hair?

Tonging

Tongs can give a number of different effects, ranging from tight curls to loose bouncy curls or spiral curls. The effect you get will depend on the size of the tong's barrel and the way you use it.

Remember to avoid **fish hooks** when you are tonging the hair. Do this by placing the tongs close to the root of the hair. Now slide them down the length of the hair to the points. Secure the ends firmly into the barrel of the tongs and then wind the hair around the barrel. Running the tongs down the length of the hair will soften the hair before it is styled and smooth down the cuticle.

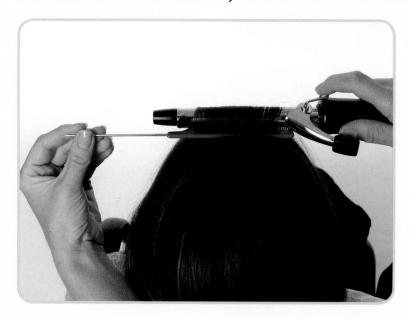

Using heated rollers

Heated rollers are used to create soft curls, lift and volume in the hair. Although they are used on dry hair, they should be placed in the hair in just the same way as the rollers you use when wet setting. For example, use a brickwork pattern or place the rollers in the direction the style will be dressed.

 Key term

Fish hooks – when the ends of the hair become bent over giving a frizzy appearance

 Top tip

When the tongs have been wound up to the scalp, make sure you place a comb between the tongs and the client's head to prevent burning the client.

 Top tip

Make sure you don't put your fingers or thumbs inside the rollers. They are very hot and will burn you.

Straightening irons

These are used to smooth and straighten the hair. They should be used to support the blow-dry and not as a lazy way to achieve straight hair!

Before starting, check you have chosen the right temperature for the type of hair you are working with (not all straighteners have this feature). This will prevent you from drying out or damaging the hair.

The hair should be sectioned and held **taut**. The straighteners are then placed near the root area and slid down the hair.

Use a comb to keep the hair smooth and untangled as the straighteners glide down the hair. You can then use the comb to support the same mesh of hair when you go over it again with the straighteners without burning your fingers.

Look back at *Follow health and safety in the salon*. Check you can remember your responsibilities when you are using electrical equipment.

Checking the balance

When you have finished, check from all angles that the style looks well balanced (in other words, not lopsided).

You should then check that the client is happy with the result and show them the back of their hair. A lot of people find it difficult to get the angle of the mirror right for this. Just remember that both you and your client are looking into the same mirror so if you can see their hair, so can they.

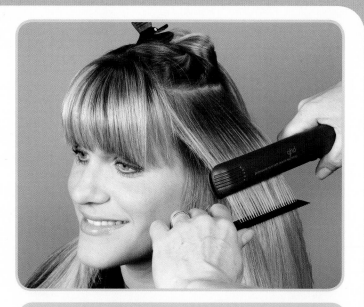

Top tip

Always use a heat protection product to protect your client's hair from the heat.

Key term

Taut – pulled straight

mirror

client

back mirror

Positioning the mirror

Try it out

Practise using the back mirror. Work with a friend to do this. Ask your friend to help you get the mirror at the right angle so that they can see the back of their hair.

Just checking

1 A fish hook can be caused when:
   a You don't use a comb when straightening the hair
   b You apply the wrong heat protection product
   c The hair the hair gets wet
   d The ends of the hair are bent over and not smoothed.

2 A heat protection product should be used before using straightening irons:
   a Because it looks professional
   b To protect the hair from the heat
   c To save you from checking the temperature of the equipment
   d If the client asks you to.

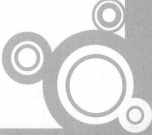

Structural hair changes and the effects of humidity

In this topic you will learn about:
- The structural changes that take place in the hair during the styling process
- How humidity affects the hair structure

When you style your hair and go out on a rainy day, have you noticed how it drops? Why do you think this happens?

Alpha and beta keratin

The styling process helps straight hair to be made curly and curly hair to be made straighter. The reason why this can happen is because of the structure of the cortex. The cortex is made up of bunches of parallel fibres and, in turn, these are made up from smaller fibres. These smaller fibres are coiled and shaped like a spiral staircase – they are called polypeptide chains. Neighbouring chains are joined together with temporary cross-linkages called hydrogen bonds. There are also links within chains.

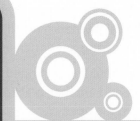

Top tip
Using styling and finishing products can help the style to last longer. They put a fine plastic coat around the hair which will help to stop the moisture getting into the hair.

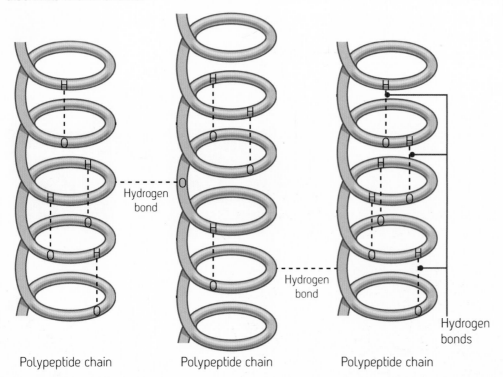

Polypeptide chain   Polypeptide chain   Polypeptide chain

Hydrogen bond

Hydrogen bond

Hydrogen bonds

It's these hydrogen bonds that give the hair its elasticity and help us to temporarily change the look of the hair (to make straight hair curly and curly hair straight). When you shampoo the hair, some of the hydrogen bonds are broken. When the hair is dried, the hydrogen bonds will reform, but often in a different place. This is why we can change the shape of the hair.

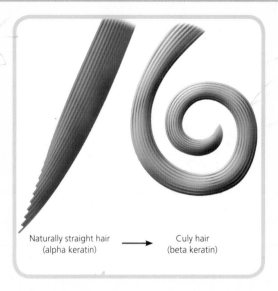

Naturally straight hair   Culy hair
(alpha keratin)   (beta keratin)

Hair that has been shampooed and left to dry naturally is described as **alpha keratin**. This is the term used for hair in its natural state. If you shampoo the hair and then set or blow-dry it into a new shape, this is called **beta keratin**.

This new shape (beta keratin) can easily be changed back to alpha keratin by wetting the hair or being in a damp atmosphere.

Using heated equipment can also break the hydrogen bonds. The equipment must be hot enough to change the water that is naturally in the hair into steam.

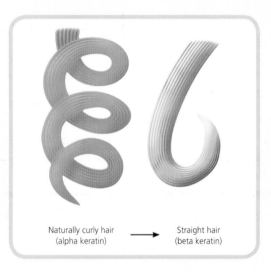

Naturally curly hair   Straight hair
(alpha keratin)   (beta keratin)

Moving from alpha to beta keratin

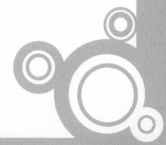

Key terms

Alpha keratin – hair that has been shampooed and left to dry naturally
Beta keratin – hair that has been shampooed and then set or blow-dried into a new shape

Humidity

'Humidity' means the amount of moisture in the air. So if it's raining, or if you are in a steamy atmosphere (for example, a bathroom), the hair will go back to its natural state of alpha keratin and the set or blow-dry will drop quickly.

Just checking

1   The hair in its new state after blow-drying is:
    a   Alpha keratin
    b   Beta keratin
    c   Gamma keratin
    d   Delta keratin.

Aftercare

Q

Why is aftercare advice important for both the client and the salon?

Aftercare advice

Before your client leaves the salon, you should give them some aftercare advice on how to keep the style looking good. This should include information about the correct products, tools and equipment that they need to use. They also need to know how they can recreate the look at home.

Talk to your client about what you are doing, and why you're doing it, throughout the service. Discuss with the client the tools and equipment you are using and ask them what type of things they have at home. Then you can explain to them how they can recreate the look. This could include advice such as making sure the airflow of the dryer is going from root to points if they're trying to achieve a smooth, shiny finish. Or you could show them how to backcomb the hair without causing any damage. All this will show your professionalism and ensure the client's hair looks good in between their visits to the salon.

When you're using products on the client's hair, explain to them what you're using and why. For example, 'I'm using a product called "thick it up" on your hair and it will make it feel and look thicker than it really is.'

You should also explain how to use the product, as many clients don't read the instructions. When the client sees that it works, they may want to buy the product so they can get the same look when they do it at home.

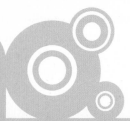

Top tip

A lot of clients have very dry and brittle hair due to overuse of heated styling equipment, such as straighteners. If you recommend a good heat protection spray it should improve the condition of their hair.

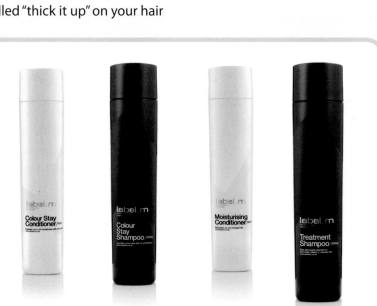

In the salon

Navin was asked to blow-dry a client for Kylie, one of the stylists, as she was running late. Kylie explained to Navin how she wanted the blow-dry done. It looked great when Navin had finished and he was really pleased. The client loved the look too. However, the following week the client returned to the salon very upset. She explained to Kylie that she'd not been able to manage her new style. Kylie explained everything to the client and she went away happy – but Kylie was not happy. She called Navin into the staffroom and told him off for not giving the client any aftercare advice. Navin tried to explain that he hadn't known the client had had a restyle but Kylie wouldn't listen.

- What went wrong? Who do you think was at fault?

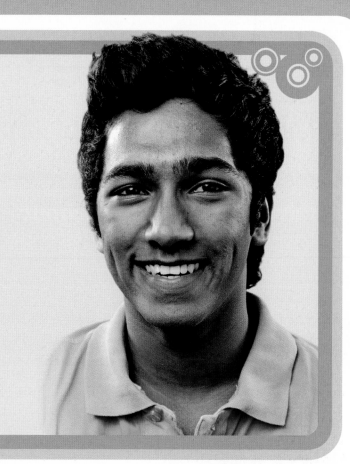

You may want to offer advice on general hair care to your client, especially if you think they may be doing something wrong. You should discuss the type of shampoo and conditioner they use at home. Ask yourself if these are the right products for the client's hair. If not, suggest something that would be right.

You could also suggest additional services at the salon such as a conditioning treatment if the hair is very dry and damaged or a cut to remove dry and damaged ends.

All of these will help to ensure the client's hair looks as good as it possibly can. The rest is up to your client!

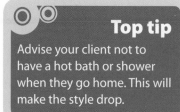

Top tip
Advise your client not to have a hot bath or shower when they go home. This will make the style drop.

Just checking
1 When chatting to the client at the end of the service, you should discuss:
   a Their forthcoming holiday
   b Where they are going that night
   c How they should maintain the look
   d What type of car they should buy.

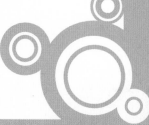

Skin care

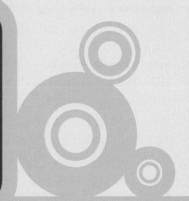

In this unit you will learn about:

- Choosing products, tools and equipment for basic skin care treatments
- Preparing yourself, the client and work area for skin care
- Recognising different skin types
- Carrying out basic skin care treatments under supervision

Introduction

A healthy glowing skin needs a good skin care routine and the right products to keep it looking clean and **blemish** free. This unit will support you while you try out skills and techniques involved in the preparation and completion of skin care treatments.

You will find out about the range of products, tools and materials needed for skin care techniques. You will also practise organising your work area and trolley with the correct items within easy reach.

You will identify the main skin types, and also learn about conditions that may stop you from carrying out treatments.

You will have the opportunity to develop professional skills while contributing to the salon's health, safety and hygiene requirements.

Top tips

- Eat a healthy balanced diet
- Sleep well
- Drink plenty of water
- Make sure you have a good skin care routine
- Never go to bed with your make-up on
- Don't pick or squeeze your spots
- Use a sunscreen and wear a hat in the sun to protect your skin
- Don't smoke, as it uses up valuable nutrients needed for healthy skin

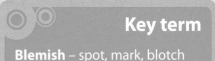

Key term

Blemish – spot, mark, blotch

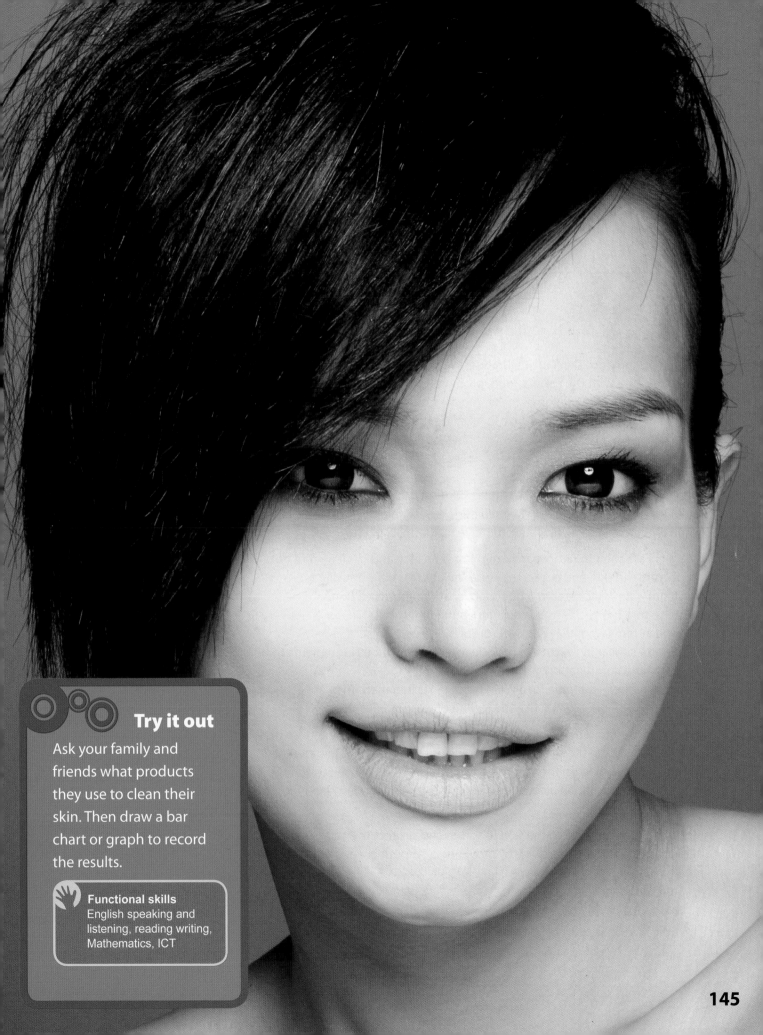

Try it out

Ask your family and friends what products they use to clean their skin. Then draw a bar chart or graph to record the results.

Functional skills
English speaking and listening, reading writing, Mathematics, ICT

145

Products, tools and equipment for skin care

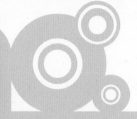

In this topic you will learn about:

- Products, tools and equipment for a basic skin care treatment

Q We spend millions on skin care products. What methods do manufacturer's use to persuade us to buy their products?

Before you carry out skin care techniques, you must first know how to set up your work area with the correct tools, products and equipment. If you visit any salon you will notice a range of these. You are going to explore many of them and the importance that they have in facial treatments.

Products

Eye make-up remover is a mild cleaning solution that helps to **dissolve** eye make-up so that it can be easily wiped off. It is available as an oil, lotion or gel. Some of them can remove waterproof eye make-up.

Cleansers are used to remove make-up from the face and to clean dirt, dust and grime from the skin and pores. They are available for different skin types:
- Cream – very thick cream is good for very dry or **mature** skin.
- Milk – thin runny cleanser is best for young or normal skin but is not very good at removing heavy or waterproof make-up.
- Lotion – similar in **texture** to milk cleansers but includes ingredients to help spotty and combination skin types.
- Facial washes – suitable for all skin types including men. They are especially popular with people that like the feeling of washing the skin.

Toners are used to remove any leftover cleanser from the skin. They also dissolve oil, refresh and cool the skin and tighten the pores. They come in different strengths depending on their ingredients and should be chosen to suit the skin type. Toners that contain alcohol are used for oily and problem skin types (these are called astringents).

Moisturisers are applied to the skin to soften and protect the surface and to help the application of make-up by providing a smooth base. As with cleansers, moisturisers are for different types:
- Creams for dry skins
- Lotions for oily skins
- Milks for young, normal or sensitive skins

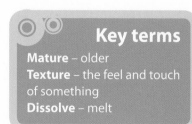

Key terms

Mature – older
Texture – the feel and touch of something
Dissolve – melt

Equipment

<u>Headband</u> – this is usually made of towelling with a **Velcro** fastening. It is used to protect a client's hair from products and stops hair from getting in the way.

<u>Gown</u> – this is used to stop the client feeling embarrassed when they remove their top clothing before a facial.

<u>Towels</u> are useful for different purposes. For example, a large towel may be used to cover the client if a blanket or duvet is not used and another medium-sized one is usually draped across the chest during the facial treatment. The amount of towels you use will depend on how your tutor tells you to set up your couch.

<u>Dampened cotton wool</u>
- Cotton wool squares are used for removing cleanser and putting on toner. They need to be large enough to wrap around two fingers.
- Half moons are cut to shape from damp cotton wool and are placed under the bottom eyelashes. They protect the skin under the eyes from the make-up that is being cleaned off.
- Circular or square eye pads are placed on the eyes during different stages of the facial treatment. They are used to shield the eyes from bright light or splashes of product that may drop into the eyes.

<u>Dry cotton wool</u> is used to cover the tip of an orange wood stick for removing make-up.

<u>Tissues</u> are usually sparated into two parts as this saves money and they also mould to the skin better. They are used to blot extra toner or moisturiser from the skin.

<u>Small plastic or metal bowls</u> hold cotton wool and tissues.

Tools

<u>Spatula</u> – this is a wide wooden stick that is used to scoop cream from pots instead of dipping fingers into creams. Using fingers is very **unhygienic** and could **contaminate** the product.

<u>Orange wood stick</u> – this is a thin wooden stick. One end is pointed and the other end is shaped like a hoof. The pointed ends are coated with cotton wool which softens the tip for safety when cleaning around the eyes. The hoof end is not used for facial treatments.

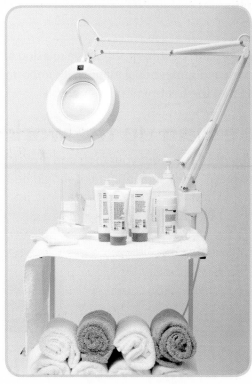

A trolley set up for facial skin care treatment

Prepare for skin care

Q Unhealthy bacteria are on every surface. Which surfaces do you think contain the most bacteria? You may be surprised at the answer. Visit the Internet to see if you can find the answer.

A skin care treatment should be relaxing and the therapist must carry it out in a calm and professional manner. It's important to prepare thoroughly beforehand so that the treatment runs smoothly.

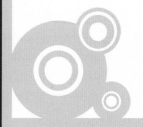

Top tips

- Don't talk too much throughout the treatment.
- Don't breathe over the client.
- Don't sniff.
- Make sure your hands and nails are smooth and not rough.
- Make sure your hands are warmed.

Setting up the work area

You need to lay out your tools and products on your trolley so that they are easy to reach. Tools and equipment should be cleaned and sterilised before use.

Equipment must be easy to reach to avoid overstretching or getting up to fetch something

Organised work area with nothing forgotten

Points to remember

Tools and equipment must be hygienic and clean before use

Work area set up – points to remember

Health, safety and hygienic working practices

Never forget how easy it is to cross-infect. Make sure that you use hygienic working practices. (Health, safety and hygiene are covered in detail in *Follow health and safety in the salon*.) Ways that you could spread bacteria are listed in the table below.

Your actions	How they could spread germs and bacteria
Not washing your hands before and after carrying out a face care treatment	Germs could be on your hands from a previous client and you could spread them to your next client.
Using fingers instead of a disposable spatula to scoop out cream from pots	The pot of cream will become a breeding ground for germs. When used, the germs will spread to people.
Blowing your nose and not washing your hands afterwards	You will have germs on your hands which you will pass to the client when you touch her face.

Client preparation

Welcome the client and introduce yourself so that she feels at ease and starts to feel confidence in you. Ask her to take a seat while you go through the client consultation.

You will need to use a record card to write down important information during the consultation. This should include:

- personal client contact details
- contra-indications or disorders of the skin and/or eyes
- skin condition and skin type
- facial products and techniques used
- your name
- date of treatment
- client signature.

Look carefully at the client's skin in a good light before you start so that you can see the skin's condition and texture. This also allows you to look for anything that may stop or **restrict** the skin care treatment from going ahead, such as a **contra-indication**. (Look back to *Anatomy and physiology* page 78 to remind yourself of possible contra-indications.) If you think that a client has a contra-indication, check with your tutor before going ahead. It is not up to you to decide whether it is safe to carry on.

Skin types

It is important that you decide on the client's skin type so that you can choose the best treatment and products to suit it. There are four main skin types:

- Normal – most common in children and teenagers. It is clear, **supple** and smooth.
- Dry – this will feel very dry to the touch. It does not shine and can feel tight due to the lack of oil.
- Oily – this skin type will look shiny and feel greasy and can have spots and blackheads.
- Combination – normal or dry but with an oily T-section down the middle (from the forehead down the nose to the chin). The oily part will look shiny.

For more information on skin types, see *Anatomy and physiology*, page 72.

Key terms

Restrict – limit
Contra-indication – a condition that may restrict or prevent a treatment being carried out
Supple – flexible, elastic

Try it out

Carry out a survey among your friends and family. Ask them what skin type they think they have. Record the results on a graph to see which skin type seems to be the most common one.

Functional skills
English speaking, reading and writing, ICT, Mathematics

Just checking

1 State two ways that bacteria could be spread from you to a client.

2 Why is it important to carry out a visual study of a client's skin?

3 What are the four main skin types?

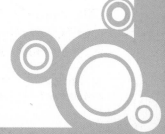

Carry out skin care

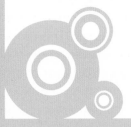

In this topic you will learn about:

- Making sure the client is comfortable before you start the treatment
- Carrying out basic skin care treatments under supervision
- Offering homecare advice

Q If a client feels comfortable throughout her treatment what positive effects could this have on her body and mind? Think of as many positive effects as you can.

Client comfort

Before you start the treatment, ask the client to remove jewellery such as dangly earrings. It is better they put it in their bag rather than place it in a bowl next to the work area. In this way, you won't be responsible if it goes missing.

Position the client on a couch, making sure they are comfortable and warm.
- Use a gown or towel to protect the client's **modesty** if necessary. Drape a towel across their chest area to protect clothing and use a headband to protect the hair from skin care products.
- Use a pillow or neck cushion if the client needs head and neck support while lying down.
- Make sure that the lighting is not too bright, the room is warm (but not too stuffy) and the atmosphere is calm.

Carry out basic skin care treatment

Make one last check of your work area, self and equipment. Check the client is comfortable and wash your hands. Now you are ready to start the treatment. This image shows a suggested cleansing routine.

Cleansing routine

1 4 strokes on chin
2 4 strokes on each cheek
3 Circles around the mouth
4 4 strokes on bridge of nose
5 4x eye circles
6 4 strokes on forehead

Key term

Modesty – possible shyness at getting undressed in front of people

Top tip

Make sure all shoes and clothes are put away so that you don't trip over them Sit down behind the couch while doing the treatment to save your legs and back from aching.

Try it out

Choose one skin care product. Look at the list of ingredients and choose two that you will find out about. For example, you could ask yourself, what do the ingredients do? Are they necessary?

 Functional skills
English reading

In the salon

It was Shabeena's turn to be the therapist in class and she was going to practise her facial techniques on Janie. However, Janie wasn't happy – she always tried to avoid being a model. The tutor had a chat with Janie about this and she eventually agreed but was very grumpy. Shabeena prepared Janie – she made sure she was comfortable and started to remove her make-up. She always wore a lot and it was caked on thickly.

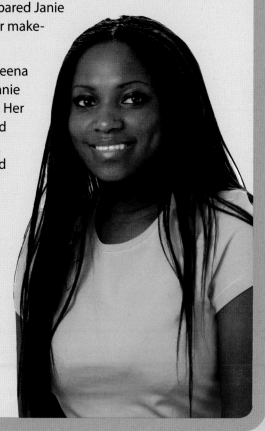

The first cleansing routine didn't clean the skin enough so Shabeena did a second and a third cleanse. It was then she realised why Janie didn't want to be a model and why she wore so much make-up. Her face was covered in spots and red blemishes and her skin looked very red and angry. Shabeena felt sorry for her and didn't really know what to do or say. The tutor came over and quietly advised Janie how she could improve her skin and what to use at home. She also told her that if she was a model more often, the facial techniques would really help her skin to improve.

Shabeena felt that this had really helped because she now had more knowledge to advise people. She had also learned how she could make clients feel at ease if they had bad skin.

- Why do you think Janie was unhappy and not cooperating with Shabeena and the tutor?
- What sort of skills do you need so that you can help clients feel at ease no matter what their skin is like?

Homecare advice

After treatment, offer your client some advice:
- Don't apply make-up for 12 hours.
- Avoid touching the skin.
- Cleanse, tone and moisturise morning and night.
- Drink plenty of water and eat a healthy diet.
- Don't touch or squeeze spots and blackheads.
- Wear a good moisturiser to protect the skin.
- Have a monthly skin care treatment.
- Protect the skin in the sun.

Just checking

1 What should the atmosphere be like to make sure the client is comfortable throughout her treatment?

2 How can you support the client's neck during the treatment?

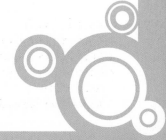

Step-by-step skin care routine

1

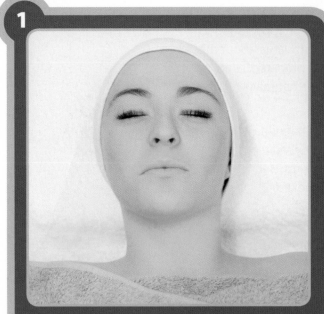

Sit client comfortably on the couch, protect her clothing and put her headband on.

2

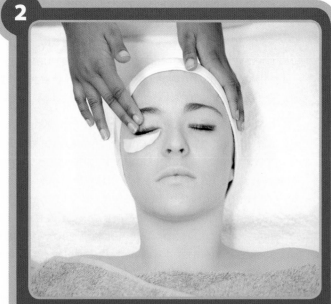

Place half moons under the bottom lashes and ask the client to close her eyes. Apply eye make-up remover in circular movements with the middle finger on the eyelids and lashes. Then remove gently with downward strokes with a clean piece of cotton wool. This will remove eyeshadow and mascara. You can use a covered orange wood stick for any stubborn make-up. Repeat if necessary.

3

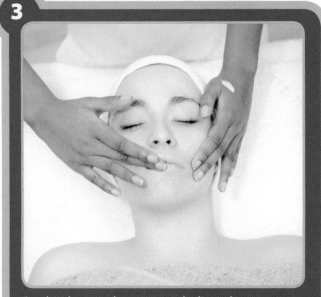

Gently rub some cleanser onto the lips, taking care not to get it in the client's mouth. With a clean piece of damp cotton wool wipe across the lips to remove the lipstick. With another piece of damp cotton wool wipe across the lips in the other direction. Support the edges of the mouth when you wipe across.

4

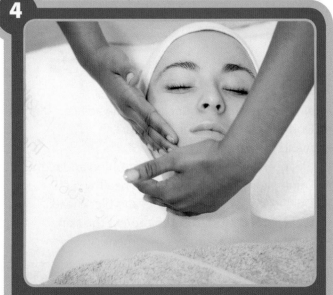

Put cleanser into the palm of your hands and press your hands over the face and neck so that you have enough product to carry out a cleansing routine. With smooth, upward strokes and movements follow a cleansing routine that your tutor gives to you or the routine on page 150. Thoroughly clean the client's skin .

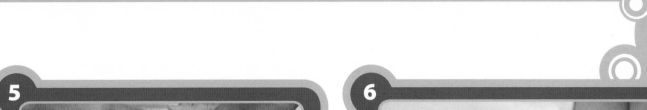

5

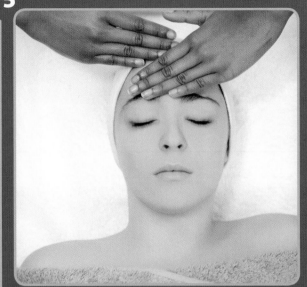

Movements should be careful and gentle. The cleanser will remove any make-up, or dirt. You will need to repeat the cleansing routine twice. Then remove the cleanser with damp cotton wool using the movements from the cleansing routine.

6

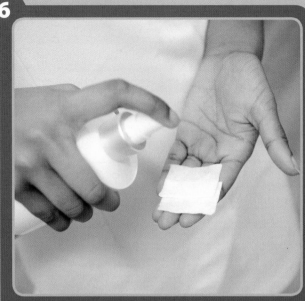

Take two pieces of damp cotton wool squares and soak them in toning lotion.

7

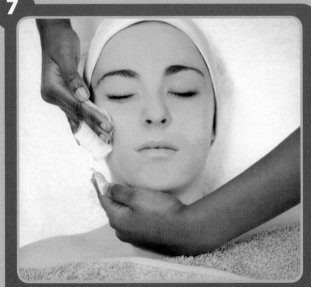

Wrap the cotton wool soaked in toner around your fingers and repeat the cleansing routine movements with the toner. This will tone the skin and remove the last traces of cleanser. Then blot the skin with a split tissue to remove any extra toner on the skin.

8

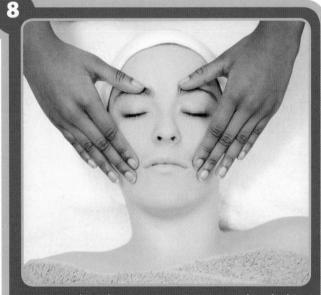

Use a spatula to decant some moisturiser and apply this evenly over the face, using the same movements as you did for the cleanser. Blot the skin with a split tissue if there is too much moisturiser on the skin.

Hand and foot care

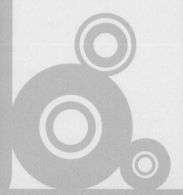

In this unit you will learn about:

- Products for hand and foot care treatments
- Equipment for hand and foot care treatments
- Preparing for hand and foot care treatments
- Identifying typical nail shapes and basic nail structure
- Factors that influence hand and foot care treatments
- Contra-indications and contra-actions
- Carrying out basic hand and foot care treatments under supervision

Introduction

Your nails can show signs of health problems in other parts of your body. Healthy nails should be a pale pink colour. If they change colour and texture, it could mean that there is a lack of vitamins, minerals or nutrients. A healthy diet will help to keep your nails healthy and attractive.

This unit will introduce you to ways that you can look after nails and surrounding skin.

Top tips

- Eat a healthy balanced diet.
- Eat foods containing calcium, zinc and vitamin D.
- Do not use your nails as tools – no picking or scraping.
- Don't bite or pick at your nails.
- Don't remove **hangnails** by pulling at them.
- Moisturise your nails and cuticles daily.
- File or trim nails regularly to keep the free edge smooth.

Key term

Hangnail – a small piece of skin or nail partly separated from the side or base of a fingernail or toenail

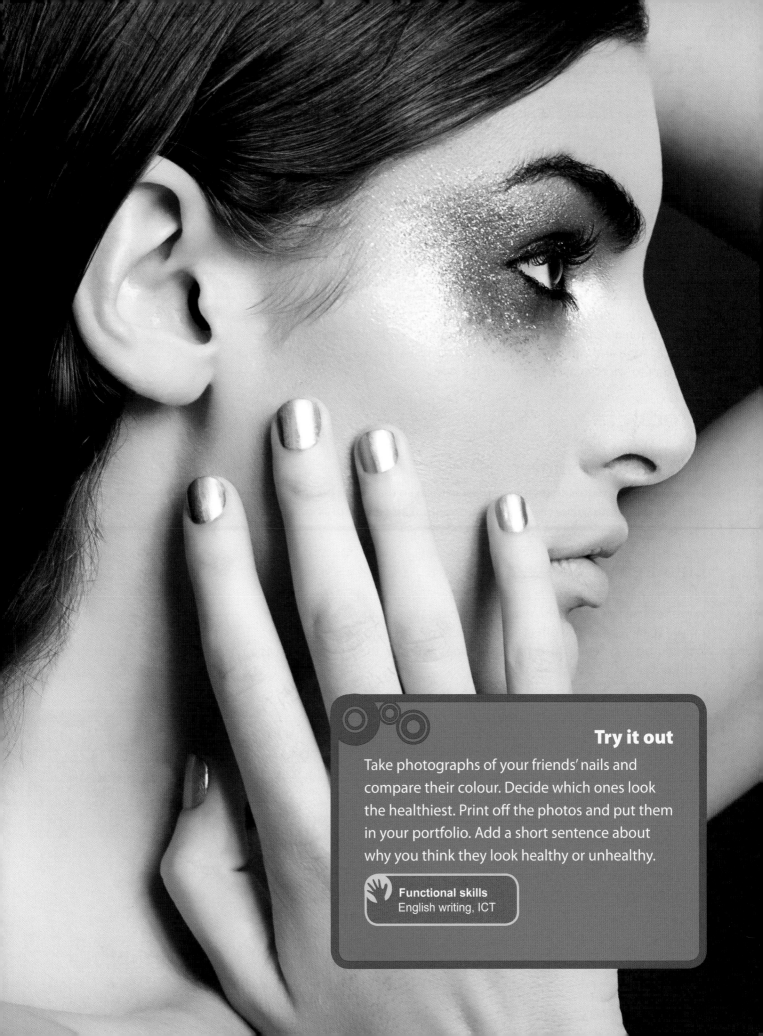

Try it out

Take photographs of your friends' nails and compare their colour. Decide which ones look the healthiest. Print off the photos and put them in your portfolio. Add a short sentence about why you think they look healthy or unhealthy.

Functional skills
English writing, ICT

Products for hand and foot care treatments

In this topic you will learn about:

- Products for hand and foot care treatments

Q Write down as many different nail products as you can think of (apart from those covered in this unit). Why might you need to use each one?

To carry out manicure and pedicure treatments, you will need a range of products, tools and equipment. Each item has a different job to do and together they work to improve the condition of the nails.

Products

Nail varnish remover

This is a chemical liquid that dissolves nail varnish so that it can be easily wiped from the **nail plate** with a piece of cotton wool. It can be very drying to the nail plate.

Coloured varnish

Nail varnishes come in a wide range of different colours and finishes. Some varnishes have a cream finish while others have special ingredients in them to give them a **pearlised effect**. Cream-effect varnish is good for nails with a lot of ridges and dents. This is because it does not show them up as much as a pearlised varnish would.

Base coat

This is usually a clear varnish that is used to stop the nail plate being stained by coloured varnish. A base coat also helps to make the varnish last longer.

Top coat

This is a clear varnish that is used on top of coloured varnish so that the colour doesn't chip or peel off as quickly. It also gives a glossy shine to the nails.

Nail strengtheners and hardeners

These are usually like clear varnishes but contain extra ingredients to provide the nails with a tough coating.

Key terms

Nail plate – the surface of the nail that covers and protects the bed of the fingernail (pink in colour)

Pearlised effect – shimmery

Top tip

Wipe around the neck of the varnish bottles after each use so that they don't become sticky and difficult to open.

Hand or foot lotion

This is used to soften and hydrate the skin towards the end of the hand or foot care treatment. It is applied using gentle massage movements, which also help to improve the blood circulation and relax the client.

Hand soak

This is a mild soapy liquid which is mixed with warm water in a bowl. The warm, soapy water softens and cleans the nails and cuticles.

Buffing paste

This is a slightly **abrasive** cream that is applied to the nail plate. The action of the cream and the **buffing tool** help to smooth out the surface of the nail plate and add natural shine.

Cuticle cream

This is a thick moisturising cream that is used to soften and nourish the cuticles. It helps to prevent the skin splitting or drying out and makes it easier to gently push back the cuticles during treatment.

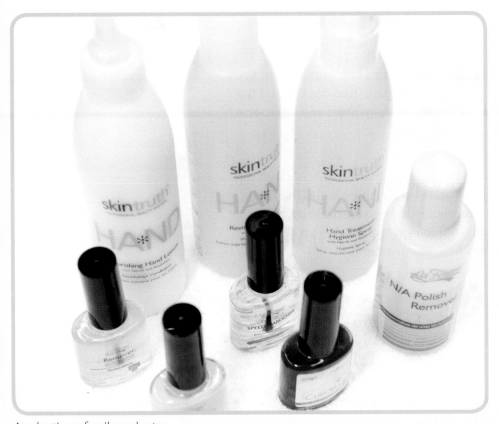

A selection of nail products

Key terms

Abrasive – rough
Buffing tool – curved tool covered in leather which is used to shine the nail plate

Top tip

Never thin out varnish with nail varnish remover. It may work the first time but it will quickly become thick again.

Try it out

In small groups, design a range of nail products. Think of a name for your brand. Then, display your designs on large posters. Be arty and creative!

Functional skills
English reading and writing, ICT

Just checking

1 What is the purpose of cuticle cream?

2 Why would you use buffing paste?

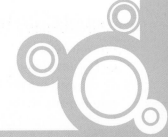

Equipment for hand and foot care treatments

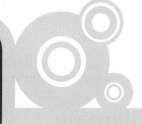

In this topic you will learn about:
- Equipment for hand and foot care treatments

Think about when you have had a hand or foot care treatment or have seen one being done. What tools and equipment were used apart from those listed in this section?

Equipment

You will need the following:

Nail file/emery board

This is used for filing and shaping the nails. Emery boards come in different sizes, widths and strengths. The coarseness of the emery board used depends on the thickness of the nails. Usually the fine side is used on fingernails and the coarse side on toenails or men's fingernails.

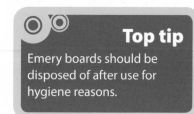

Top tip

Emery boards should be disposed of after use for hygiene reasons.

Orange wood sticks

These are used for cleaning under the nail and also for cuticle work. They are tipped with cotton wool. When the cotton wool has been used it must be replaced with a clean piece. The cotton wool softens the wooden tip, which stops the cuticles and skin becoming sore during treatment.

Spatulas

These are made from wood or plastic and are used for scooping out cream or lotion from pots hygienically.

Gown

A gown is used to protect the client's clothing from splashes or spills during a treatment.

Towels

You will need at least two towels so that you are able to dry feet and hands after they have been soaked in warm soapy water. Also towels can be placed on the client's lap to protect their clothing and soak up any splashes of water.

A selection of nail tools

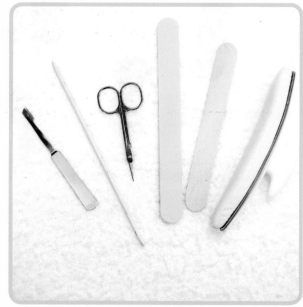

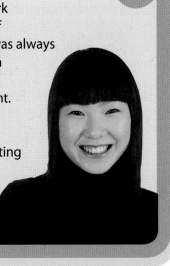
Cotton wool

Cotton wool should be shaped into small balls and placed in a bowl. They will be used throughout hand and foot care treatments. They are used with nail varnish remover to remove varnish from the nail plate. They are also used to cover the end of an orange wood stick when applying cuticle cream and cleaning under the nail.

Tissues

You will need several of these. They are used to wipe products from the client's nails. They can also be tucked into the ends of sleeves or trouser legs to stop creams staining the client's clothes.

Manicure/finger bowl

This is usually a specially shaped gripper bowl with a lid that has a small hole in it for the thumb and a larger hole for the rest of the fingers. The lid prevents water spills and can be easily removed for thorough cleaning. It is filled with warm soapy water to soak the client's hands during the manicure.

Pedicure bowl

This may be a simple plastic bowl or a foot-shaped bowl. Some salons have foot spas which massage the feet while they are soaking in the water.

Dish or bowl

You will need one bowl for the cotton wool balls and another for the tissues.

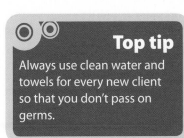

Top tip

Always use clean water and towels for every new client so that you don't pass on germs.

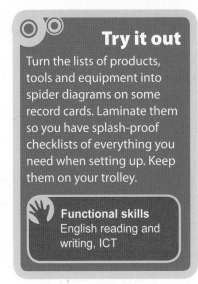

Try it out

Turn the lists of products, tools and equipment into spider diagrams on some record cards. Laminate them so you have splash-proof checklists of everything you need when setting up. Keep them on your trolley.

Functional skills
English reading and writing, ICT

Just checking

1 Give two uses of an orange wood stick in nail care treatments.

2 Describe what a manicure/finger bowl looks like.

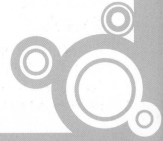

Preparation for hand and foot care

In this topic you will learn about:

- Preparation of yourself, your client and your work area for hand and foot care treatments
- Following safe and hygienic working practices
- Communicating and acting in a professional manner

Q How many nail diseases and disorders can be caused by using unclean tools and incorrectly using them? Make a list of them.

Successful nail treatments depend on good organisation of your work area and careful client care and consultation. Client consultations are important so that you can check whether there are any contra-indications that may stop the treatment or will require you to **adapt** it. You also need to know what the client's needs are so that you can plan your treatment techniques.

Setting up your work area

On pages 158–59 you learned about the various things you need for a hand or foot care treatment. Remind yourself what they are and set up your work area by laying them out in an organised way.

Choosing your products, techniques, tools and equipment will also depend on influencing factors. These are covered on page 164.

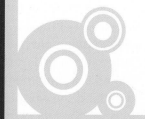

Key term

Adapt – change the way to do something

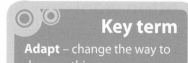

Top tip

Personal hygiene and appearance is important at all times during your preparation and treatment. In addition, if you look the part, you are more likely to feel confident and professional.

Check tools and equipment are clean and hygienic → Check work area is sanitised → Check towels are laundered → Check new sheets of protective tissue/couch roll are used for each client ↓

Check your hair is tied back and you are clean and tidy ← Check your hands and nails are clean ← Check lined waste bin is nearby to immediately throw away waste

Client preparation

Always remember that it is important to act well and communicate in a positive way with your clients and colleagues. Further information on this can be found in *Presenting a professional image in a salon*.

Welcome the client and introduce yourself so that they feel at ease and have confidence in you. Ask them to take a seat while you go through a few questions for your records.

Use a record card to write down client information. It is important to keep a record of clients and their treatments. You will need to be very respectful and ask questions in a quiet and confidential manner. Client information will include:

- personal client contact details
- the treatment they will be having
- nail varnish colour
- contra-indications or disorders of the nail
- nail and skin condition and nail shape
- your name
- date of treatment
- client signature.

Before you begin any treatment, ask the client to remove their jewellery and place it in their bag. It is much better if they keep it safe rather than putting it in a bowl next to the work area. In this way, you won't be responsible if it goes missing.

Top tip

Remember – positive communication and behaviour is important during every stage of the treatment, including the consultation.

Try it out

Search for photographs of nail diseases and disorders on the Internet and print them off. Cut them out and stick them onto small cards. Write the name of the disease/disorder next to each one. Use these cards to help you recognise them.

Functional skills
English reading and writing, ICT

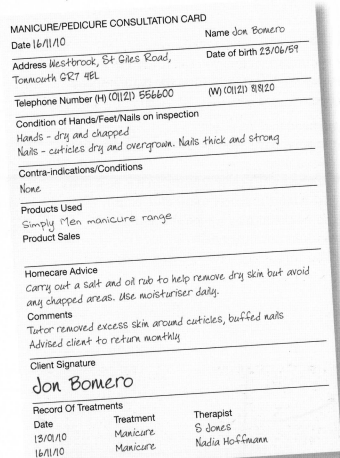

MANICURE/PEDICURE CONSULTATION CARD

Date 16/11/10   Name Jon Bomero

Address Westbrook, St Giles Road, Tonmouth GR7 4EL   Date of birth 23/06/59

Telephone Number (H) (0121) 556600   (W) (0121) 818120

Condition of Hands/Feet/Nails on inspection
Hands – dry and chapped
Nails – cuticles dry and overgrown. Nails thick and strong

Contra-indications/Conditions
None

Products Used
Simply Men manicure range
Product Sales

Homecare Advice
Carry out a salt and oil rub to help remove dry skin but avoid any chapped areas. Use moisturiser daily.

Comments
Tutor removed excess skin around cuticles, buffed nails
Advised client to return monthly

Client Signature
Jon Bomero

Record Of Treatments

Date	Treatment	Therapist
13/01/10	Manicure	S Jones
16/11/10	Manicure	Nadia Hoffmann

A consultation card for a manicure or pedicure

Just checking

1 Why is it important to maintain your personal hygiene and appearance during your preparation?

2 List two things that you need to record on the client's record card (specific to nail treatments).

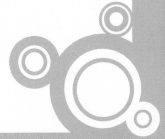

Nail shapes and nail structure

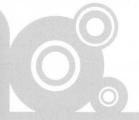

In this topic you will learn about:
- Nail shapes
- Nail structure

What do you think is the most common nail shape? Try to find out by looking at your friends' and/or colleagues' nail shapes.

Shaping the nails

Before you carry out a treatment it is important that you can recognise the client's nail shape. They vary from one client to another and the natural shape normally mirrors the line of the cuticle.

When shaping the client's nails you need to think about:
- the client's job and lifestyle – they may have a job where they use their hands a lot (for example, gardening or cleaning)
- what the client wants – it may not be a practical shape and so it is best to try to encourage the client to choose a more practical shape and length
- the current shape of the nail – some clients may want a shape that isn't possible for the natural shape and length of their nails

Top tip
Nail shapes should suit the person, their job and their lifestyle. Make sure you give a client a shape that is practical.

Fingernail shapes

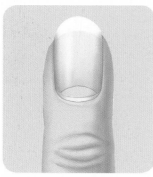

Oval – this is practical and flatters the appearance of the hands. It makes the fingers look longer and is quite hardwearing because of its smooth edges.

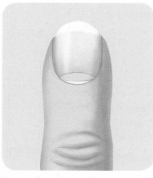

Round – this is also very practical, hardwearing and strong. But it is not very flattering.

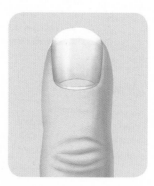

Square – this shape is less likely to break and is hardwearing. It is ideal for manual workers, typists and medical staff.

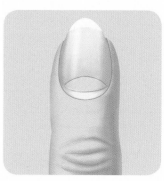

Pointed – this shape is the weakest. Filing into the sides of the nail weakens it. It is best not to file a client's nails in this way, even though the client may think that it makes the nails look longer.

Toenail shapes

These are best kept naturally square with any rough edges smoothed with an emery board. The toenails should be cut straight across with nail scissors. Your tutor will need to do this. Filing toenails into the corners can cause ingrown toenails.

Nail structure

Look back at pages 76–77 in *Anatomy and physiology* for information on basic nail structure.

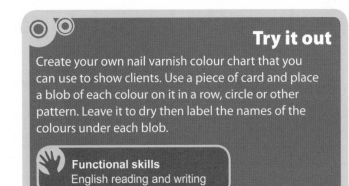

Try it out

Create your own nail varnish colour chart that you can use to show clients. Use a piece of card and place a blob of each colour on it in a row, circle or other pattern. Leave it to dry then label the names of the colours under each blob.

Functional skills
English reading and writing

In the salon

Shabeena really enjoyed practising nail care treatments on clients. However, she still needed to concentrate carefully on getting the routine in the correct order.

One day, a client brought in her own nail varnish. Because Shabeena didn't have to follow the step where the client chose the colour at the start, she was thrown from her routine. When it got to the final varnishing part, she forgot to help the client on with her jewellery and coat as well as forgetting to tell the client it was best to wait until the nails were quite dry before doing these things. When she realised, she panicked – all the client's nails were smudged. She was very upset but her tutor explained that it was a good lesson to learn from. As she grew more confident with the routine, she wouldn't get so flustered!

Shabeena's motto now is 'all mistakes are a lesson that you can learn by'.

- Do you agree? Can you think of any mistakes you have learned from?

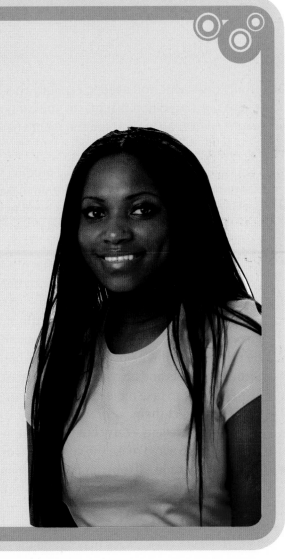

Just checking

1 List three fingernail shapes.

2 How should you shape a toenail?

3 Which fingernail shape is the least practical?

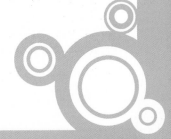

Factors that could influence treatment

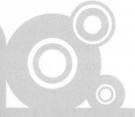

In this topic you will learn about:
- Factors influencing hand and foot care treatments

Q Why do you think that so many people now choose to have artificial nail extensions rather than natural nails? Think of all the different reasons why this might be.

Before any treatment, you need to carefully check the nails and the skin around them. You might see a condition that means you cannot carry out the treatment. Alternatively, you might need to adapt it to suit the client's nails and skin.

Factors include:
- Allergies – if the client is allergic to a product that you use, this could cause inflammation and redness. It could even make the condition worse.
- Nail length – if the nails are long and need to be cut or filed, this will affect the time it will take you to do the hand care treatment. It can also be more difficult to varnish the nails when they are long.
- Skin condition – dry skin will need richer moisturisers and cuticle creams. Ingredients such as nail varnish remover, or the hands being left in the water bowl too long, can make the dryness worse.
- Nail condition – some nails are very **brittle** and not very flexible, which means they can break easily. It is better to choose a nail shape such as an oval or square when you file them, as this helps to prevent nail breakage.
- Surrounding cuts and abrasions – these can sting if products get into them during the treatment, so take more care around these areas. You could cover them with a plaster to protect them.
- Bruising and swelling – carry out your treatment gently around any areas of bruising and swelling to avoid make the condition worse or hurting the client.
- Severe nail damage – it is better not to continue a treatment if the client has severe nail damage unless it is only on one nail, is not due to a nail disease and is covered up.
- Client expectations – most clients have an idea of what they want from a treatment. For example, the colour they want their nails painted and the length and shape of them. However, their choice may not be the most suitable, so try to encourage a client to decide on the best colour, shape and products for their skin and nails.

To find out whether any of these will influence the treatment, look (a visual study) at the skin and nails before you start. Feeling the hands or feet (a manual check) is also useful as it will help you to decide on the condition of the skin.

The visual study and manual check also allow you to check for any **contra-indications** that may prevent or **restrict** the hand or foot care treatment.

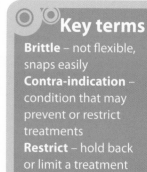

Key terms
Brittle – not flexible, snaps easily
Contra-indication – condition that may prevent or restrict treatments
Restrict – hold back or limit a treatment

Look (visual study)

Before you can complete all the details on the record card (such as disorders, contra-indications, condition and shape of nails) look carefully at the fronts and backs of the client's hands, nails and surrounding skin. For a pedicure, look at the tops and soles of the feet, toenails and surrounding skin. Before you do this, use a **sanitising spray** or gel to clean yours and your client's hands or feet. Then remove any varnish from the nails so that you can see the natural nail clearly.

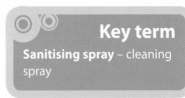

Key term

Sanitising spray – cleaning spray

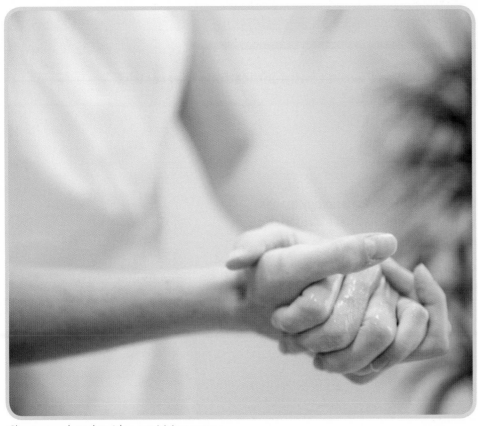

Clean your hands with a sanitising spray or gel before you begin a service

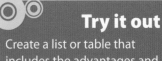

Try it out

Create a list or table that includes the advantages and disadvantages of natural nails compared to artificial nail extensions. You will have to ask lots of different people – old, young, male and female – so that you can create a complete list.
Then gather the results and turn them into a graph.

Functional skills
English speaking, reading and writing, ICT, Mathematics

Top tip

Feeling the condition of the skin and nails will help you plan the products and techniques the client will benefit from.

Feel (manual check)

Next use your hands and fingertips to feel the skin and nails of the client.

- Is the skin soft and smooth or dry and flaky?
- Are the nails smooth or do they have ridges?
- Are the cuticles rough or smooth?

Just checking

1 What are you looking for when you check over the client's nails and hands?

2 When you do a manual check of the client's nails and surrounding skin, what sort of things are you looking for?

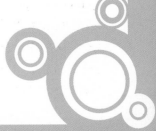

Contra-indications and contra-actions

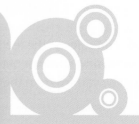

In this topic you will learn about:

- Contra-indications
- Contra-actions

Q What are the safest ways to avoid contra-indications that restrict hand/foot and nail treatments?

Contra-indications

Contra-indications are covered in detail in *Anatomy and physiology* (pages 80–81). It is essential that you are aware that a client may have a **restricting contra-indication** or one that may prevent treatment.

Any of the following could be a sign of a contra-indication. If you see any of these you must check with your tutor before continuing.

Look for:

- any signs of redness or swelling
- any signs of nail **discolouration**
- any signs of yellowing on or under the nails
- cuts, **abrasions**, swelling or lumps.

> ### Key terms
>
> **Restricting contra-indications** – contra-indications that need to be worked around
> **Discoloration** – stain or mark
> **Abrasions** – scratches

Contra-actions

These are unwanted conditions that may happen during or after a hand or foot care treatment. They may be just annoying or they could cause pain or soreness. Contra-actions that could happen include:

- Erythema – this is redness of the skin caused by an increase in blood circulation to the area. It is completely normal if it is very mild and has happened after a hand and arm massage. However, if the area is very red it may be a sign of soreness, injury or an allergy.
- Irritation – a product or technique may cause itching or irritation to the area. This could be a sign that it is not suitable for the client or that she is allergic to it.
- Swelling – this shouldn't happen during or after a hand or foot care treatment and could be a sign of soreness, injury or allergy.

If your client shows any signs of a contra-action during treatment you must stop immediately, remove the product and report it to your supervisor. After this you may apply a soothing lotion that your supervisor has agreed is safe to use.

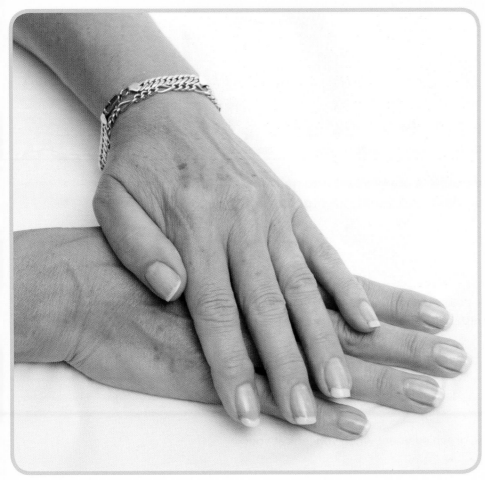

Being aware of the effects of contra-indications and contra-actions will help make sure your treatment is successful

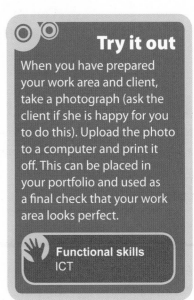

Try it out

When you have prepared your work area and client, take a photograph (ask the client if she is happy for you to do this). Upload the photo to a computer and print it off. This can be placed in your portfolio and used as a final check that your work area looks perfect.

Functional skills
ICT

Just checking

1 What is a contra-indication?

2 What is a contra-action?

Carry out hand and foot care treatments

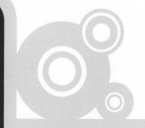

In this topic you will learn about:

- Carrying out basic hand and foot care treatments under supervision
- Aftercare advice

Q **Can you find out how many years ago nail treatments became popular? How have treatments changed over the years?**

Before you start

Now you are prepared, here are some points to remember before you start:

- Ask the client to choose a nail varnish before you start the treatment so that it saves time later.
- Before you varnish the nails, offer to help the client with putting their jewellery and coat back on
- Advise clients to wear open-toed sandals or flip flops to avoid smudging toenails.

At the end, you will have a great sense of achievement when you look at your finished work.

Top tip

If you have a paying client, ask them to pay before you start so that they don't smudge their nails at the end.

Hand and foot massage

At the end of a hand or foot care treatment, a foot or hand massage can be carried out. Cream or lotion is applied to the client's hands or feet. This will soften the skin and improve circulation to the skin and nails, which will improve the colour of the skin and encourage the growth of the nails. Massage is also a very relaxing and enjoyable end to the treatment for the client.

Your tutor will show you a basic hand and foot massage using **effleurage** and **petrissage** massage movements, which you can then practise yourself. Refer to the images on page 173 for some effleurage and petrissage massage movements that are used during the massage routine.

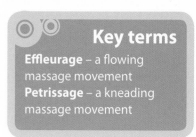

Key terms

Effleurage – a flowing massage movement
Petrissage – a kneading massage movement

Step-by-step hand care

You will complete this routine on both hands.

1

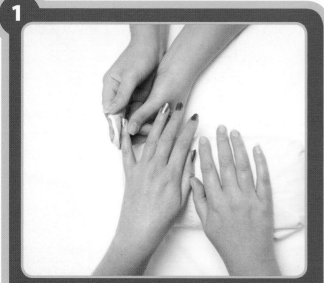

Clean each nail with a piece of cotton wool soaked in nail varnish remover. Hold it for a few seconds and then wipe down the nail. This will remove the varnish without the need to rub. Clean around the cuticles with a cotton wool covered orange wood stick with remover. This should remove any staining.

2

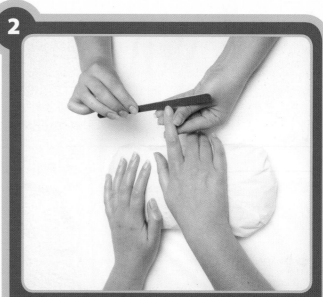

Using the fine side of the emery board, use a side-to-centre filing action. Do not use a sawing action, as this may cause the nails to split. File away any rough edges and shape the nails.

3

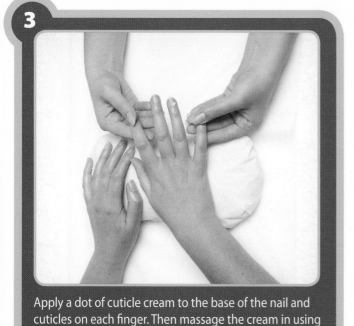

Apply a dot of cuticle cream to the base of the nail and cuticles on each finger. Then massage the cream in using circular movements with your thumbs.

4

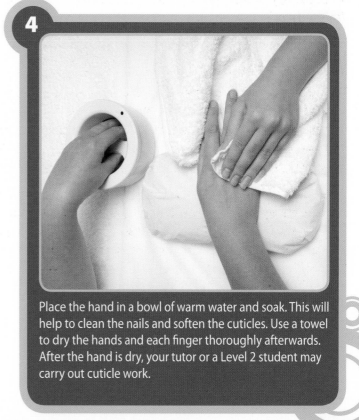

Place the hand in a bowl of warm water and soak. This will help to clean the nails and soften the cuticles. Use a towel to dry the hands and each finger thoroughly afterwards. After the hand is dry, your tutor or a Level 2 student may carry out cuticle work.

5

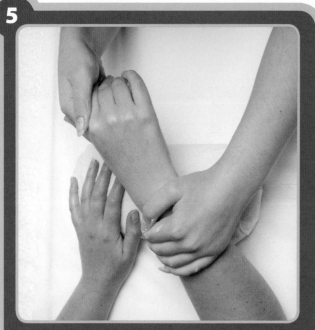

Apply the hand cream using smooth stroking movements. The cream will soften and smooth the skin and nails and relax the client. You can follow the massage advice on page 173.

6

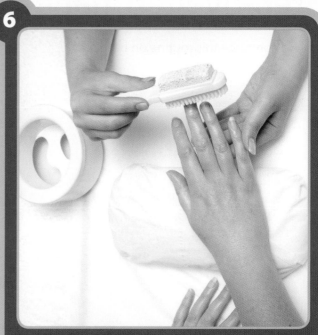

With warm soapy water, gently wash the nails with a soft brush to remove any grease from the massage. Put a small dot of buffing paste onto the centre of each nail. Use your buffing tool to stroke gently but firmly down the nail, from base to free edge. Don't buff each nail more than four times as it could weaken them. If your client prefers her nails to be buffed instead of varnished, carry this out now.

7

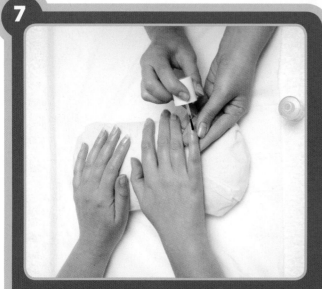

If the nails are going to be varnished, remove the hand cream from the surface of each nail by wiping them with cotton wool soaked in varnish remover. Then apply a suitable base coat.

8

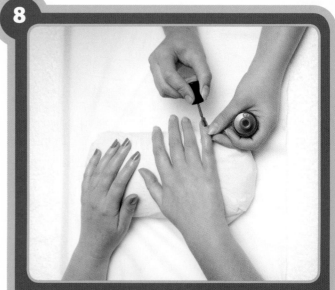

Varnish should be applied in thin strokes. Try to only do four strokes for each nail and take care not to go into the cuticles and surrounding skin. Support the client's hand while holding the nail varnish bottle and complete the strokes with your other hand. (See nail painting instructions on page 172).

Step-by-step foot care

You will complete this routine on both feet.

1

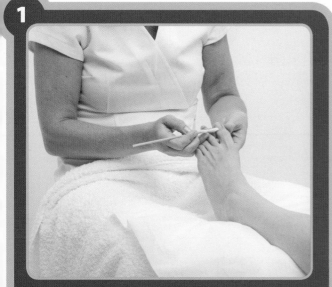

Clean each nail with a piece of cotton wool soaked in nail varnish remover. Hold it for a few seconds and then wipe down the nail. This will remove the varnish without the need to rub. Clean around the cuticles with a cotton wool covered orange wood stick with remover. This should remove any staining.

2

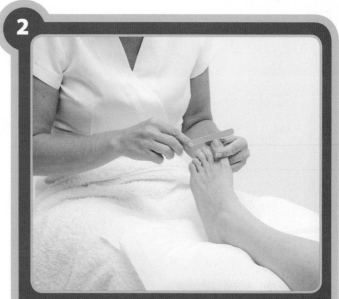

Ask your tutor to cut the nails straight across if they need it. Then, using the coarse side of the emery board, use a side-to-centre filing action. File away any rough edges and shape the nails straight across to prevent ingrowing toenails.

3

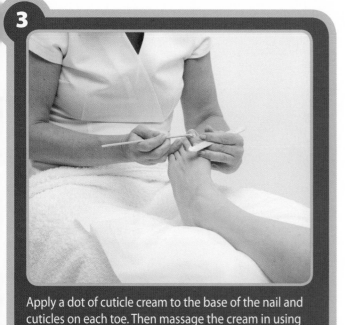

Apply a dot of cuticle cream to the base of the nail and cuticles on each toe. Then massage the cream in using circular movements with your thumbs.

4

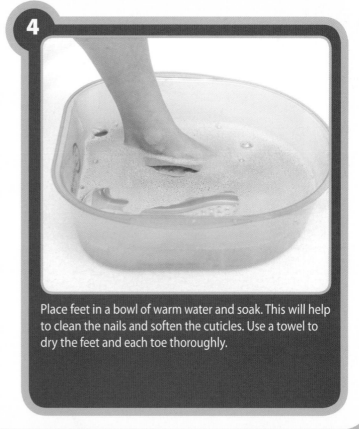

Place feet in a bowl of warm water and soak. This will help to clean the nails and soften the cuticles. Use a towel to dry the feet and each toe thoroughly.

5

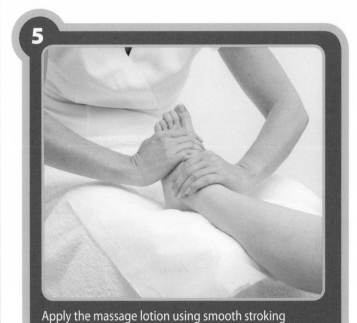

Apply the massage lotion using smooth stroking movements. The cream will soften and smooth the skin and nails and relax the client. You can follow the massage advice on page 173.

6

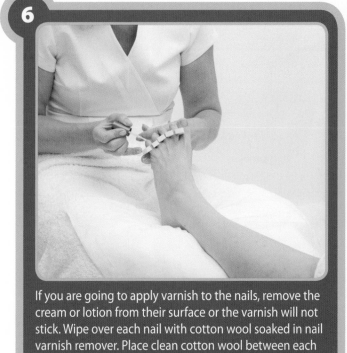

If you are going to apply varnish to the nails, remove the cream or lotion from their surface or the varnish will not stick. Wipe over each nail with cotton wool soaked in nail varnish remover. Place clean cotton wool between each toe so that they do not smudge when they are varnished. (See nail painting instructions below.)

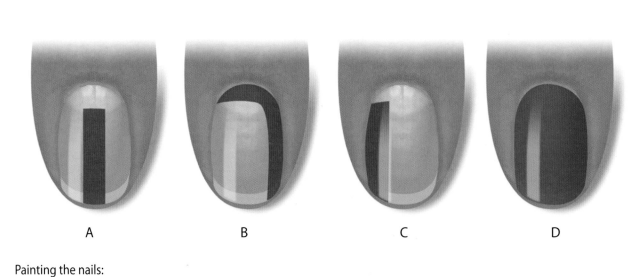

A   B   C   D

Painting the nails:
a) begin with one central application
b) then apply the varnish to the right
c) then apply the varnish to the left
d) go over the whole nail to smooth the varnish.

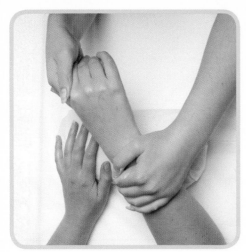

Effleurage massage movements on the hands

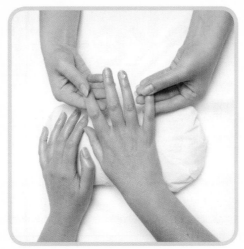

Petrissage massage movements on the hands

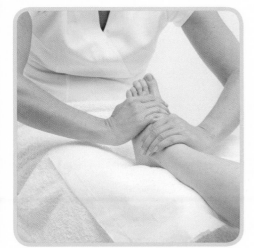

Effleurage massage movements on the feet

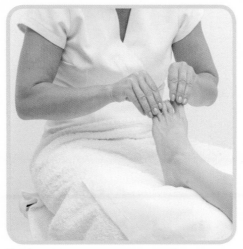

Petrissage massage movements on the feet

Aftercare advice

- Wear rubber gloves when washing up and gardening gloves to protect the skin and nails.
- Don't use nails to scrape or open things. This will weaken them.
- Don't pick at nails and cuticles if there is a rough bit. Use cream to soften or a file to get rid of any rough edges to the nail.
- Apply moisturiser to hands and feet daily to keep the skin soft.
- Don't go bare footed or hard skin will build up on the feet.
- Try to make time for a pedicure once a month and a manicure every two weeks.
- Avoid wearing high-heeled shoes for too long.

Just checking

1 List three pieces of aftercare advice that you could give to your client.

2 What is the purpose of hand and foot massage at the end of a treatment?

Basic make-up application

In this unit you will learn about:

- Equipment tools and products for make-up including how and when to use them
- Factors that could influence make-up
- Different skin types
- Preparation of yourself, your client and work area for make-up
- Applying and removing basic make-up application under supervision

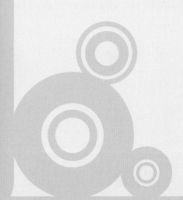

Introduction

Make-up is an art form and allows you to be creative. Using different colours and techniques to **enhance** a client's best features are valuable skills. Many people wear make-up – it is as popular now as ever and follows fashion trends and styles.

This unit will help you to develop these skills so that you can apply make-up using a variety of tools, products, colours and techniques.

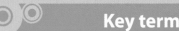

Top tips

- Always apply make-up to clean, moisturised skin.
- Always remove make-up before you go to bed.
- Don't blow on make-up brushes as this will make them unhygienic.
- Buy a good set of make-up brushes. It will make a big difference to the finished result.

Key term

Enhance – improve, make more attractive

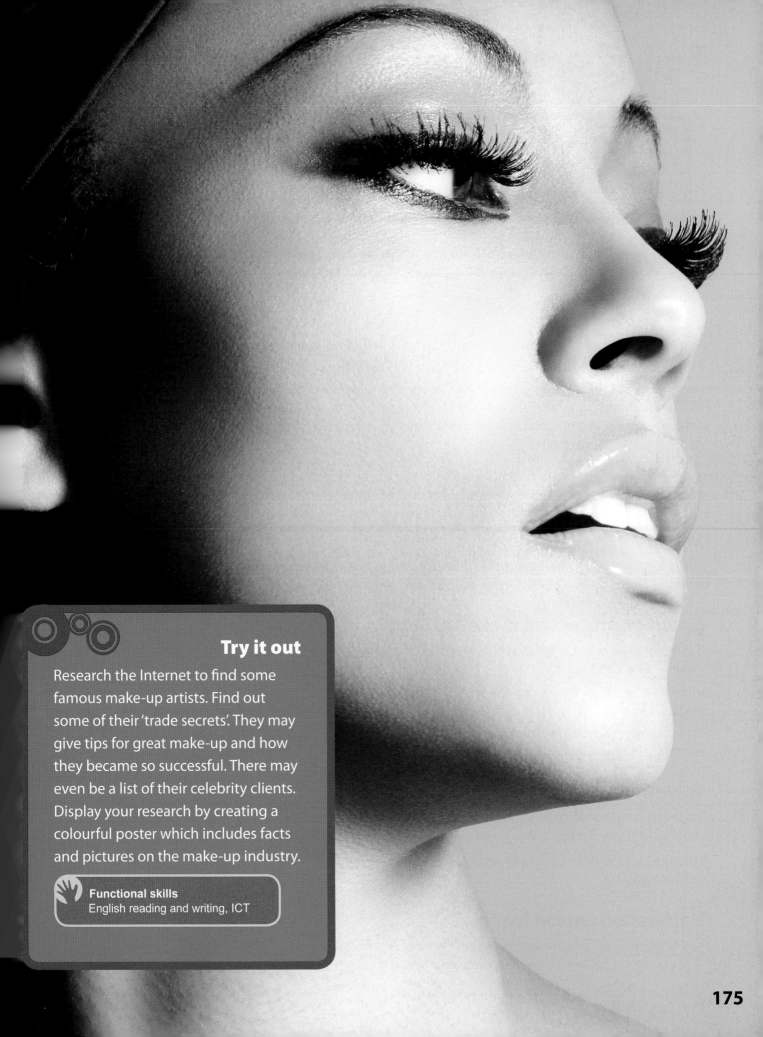

Try it out

Research the Internet to find some famous make-up artists. Find out some of their 'trade secrets'. They may give tips for great make-up and how they became so successful. There may even be a list of their celebrity clients. Display your research by creating a colourful poster which includes facts and pictures on the make-up industry.

Functional skills
English reading and writing, ICT

Equipment for make-up

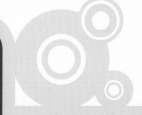

Research how much a make-up artist gets paid each day for fashion and media work. Do you think it's well paid?

To be able to carry out make-up application you must first know how to set up your work area with the correct tools, products and equipment.

From make-up brushes and mixing palettes to amazing colours and products, all of these things will be needed so that you can create a professional look. The tools, equipment and products are sold from beauty counters in department stores, salons and pharmacies.

Equipment

Mirror

This is to allow the client to look at the make-up that has been applied. She can do this at stages throughout the application as well as at the end.

Gown or protective make-up cape

A gown or make-up cape is used to protect the client's clothing during the make-up application.

Headband

This is usually made of towelling with a Velcro fastening and is used to protect a client's hair from products. It also stops hair getting in the way.

Towels

These are useful for different purposes. For example, you can protect the client's clothing with one if there is not a gown or make-up cape available.

The amount of towels you use will depend on how your tutor tells you to set up for your make-up.

Dampened cotton wool

- Cotton wool squares are used for removing cleanser and putting on toner. They need to be large enough to wrap around two fingers.

Key term

Decant – empty out a small amount of product from a pot or tube onto a spatula or palette

Top tip

When using any make-up, don't use it straight from the pot. You must first **decant** the product onto a spatula or other suitable tool and then work from this.

- Half moons – these are cut to shape from damp cotton wool. They are placed under the bottom eyelashes to protect the skin under the eyes from the make-up that is being cleaned off.

Dry cotton wool

This is used to cover the tip of an orange wood stick for removing make-up.

Tissues

Tissues are usually split in two as this saves money and they also mould to the skin better. They are used to blot extra toner or moisturiser from the skin.

Bowls

Small plastic or metal bowls are needed to hold cotton wool and tissues.

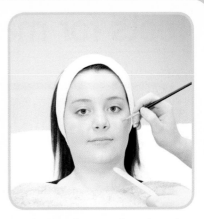

Decant products and apply with a brush

In the salon

Naima left college with an NVQ Level 2 in Beauty Therapy. She started work as a mobile therapist specialising in manicures and make-up. She visited people in their homes when they wanted treatments for special occasions or weddings.

After 18 months she realised that she wanted to become a make-up artist for runway shows and model agencies. She had taken photographs of all the make-up looks she had done and displayed them in a portfolio. She took it to an interview for a course in fashion and photographic make-up. The one-year course was during the evenings so she could continue to earn while she learned.

During the course she made a few contacts with model agencies and completed work experience on a few photo shoots. One of the agencies was so impressed with her portfolio, hard work and excellent make-up skills that they offered to put her on their books. They said they would contact her when they needed an extra make-up artist.

It wasn't a full-time position so Naima needed to carry on with bridal make-ups to earn money. However, she was gradually getting media work, building her skills and her reputation. It was hard work and very competitive but her aim was to become one of the first make-up artists that people called on for a job, not the extra one!

- What skills do you think you need for a career in make-up? In what other ways could you progress and follow a career in media and photographic make-up?

Try it out

Visit www.pearsonhotlinks. co.uk for a list of websites covering some of the big names in the make-up industry. Enter the express code P7511. Use these websites to find out about some of the tools and products available for make-up. You should also pick up some tips and tricks of the make-up trade. Print off and cut out some of the photos and pictures and use as the front cover of your make-up evidence folder.

Functional skills
English reading, ICT

Just checking

1 Why shouldn't you scoop out cream from pots using your fingers?

2 Why should you split the tissues before use?

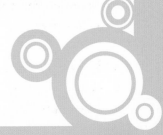

Tools for make-up

Q Make-up brushes vary a great deal in price and quality. Can you find out what the brushes are made from and how this affects the price charged for them?

Tools

You need to know about make-up tools so that you can achieve the look that you and your client are aiming for.

Brushes – the tools of the trade

You will need different brushes for each stage of make-up application. A good set of brushes that is well looked after and cleaned properly will last you a long time.

If you use good quality brushes, you will get a more natural and longer lasting look. You will also have greater control of your make-up techniques.

The brushes included with most make-up kits are simply not good enough. They are usually poor quality blush brushes and too small and coarse to apply make-up properly. This is why you see some people with blotchy, uneven make-up.

If you have a small budget, start with just three or four basic brushes – blusher, eyeliner, eyebrow and shadow. Then add on from there.

Here is a selection of tools and brushes that are most commonly used.

Top tip

Do not re-dip brushes into make-up after you have used them on the client's face, eyes or lips. It's unhygienic.

Type of brush	What it looks like	What it's used for
Powder brush	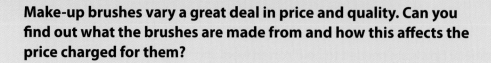	A soft oversized brush for applying pressed or loose powder application
Blusher brush	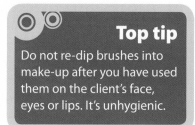	A tapered brush on both sides that allows for perfect blending

Fluff brush		This brush blends all your eyeshadow colours to give a natural look
Eyeliner brush		A small brush, rounded to a point, designed to give a perfect line every time – apply wet or dry
Lip brush		For the application of lip colour
Small sponge		Used in the application of eyeshadow. You get more coverage with this than if you apply eye colour with a brush
Brow lash brush		A duo brush used to comb clumpy lashes and unruly eyebrows

Disposable applicators

You will need a variety of disposable brushes such as mascara, lip and eyeliner. This is for hygiene reasons. The brushes usually come in packs of 50 and can be thrown away immediately after use.

Palette

This is circular and flat and can be used to mix make-up colours. It is especially useful when you are mixing foundation and lipstick or lip gloss colours. You can also put products on the palette after you have decanted them from their pot.

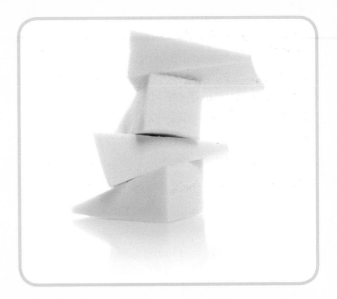

Sponges

Make-up sponges are usually made of latex and triangular in shape. They are shaped this way to make it easier to apply foundation in the curves, dips and narrow parts of the face.

Just checking

1 Name three different make-up brushes.

2 What is the purpose of disposable make-up brushes?

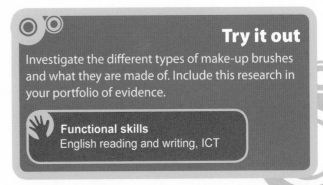

Try it out

Investigate the different types of make-up brushes and what they are made of. Include this research in your portfolio of evidence.

Functional skills
English reading and writing, ICT

Products for make-up (1)

In this topic you will learn about:

- Skin cleansing products including how and when to use them

Q Many skin care products sold today are hypo-allergenic. What does this mean and how does it help the skin?

Skin cleansing products

Product	Purpose	Information	When to use	How to use
Eye make-up remover	To clean off eye make-up	Available as an oil, lotion or gel – some remove waterproof make-up	Before make-up application	Use damp cotton wool squares and/or cotton buds to gently clean around the eyes and on the eyelashes.
Cleansers	To remove make-up on the face and to clean dirt, dust and grime from the skin and pores	Available in different types for different skins (see *Skin care*, page 146)	After eye make-up removal, before toner	Use damp cotton wool squares and follow the cleansing routine from *Skin care*, page 152.
Toners	To remove any leftover cleanser from the skin. They also dissolve oil, refresh and cool the skin and tighten the pores.	Available in different types for different skins	After cleansing and before moisturiser	Apply with damp cotton wool squares, following the same routine used to clean the face.
Moisturiser	Applied to the skin to soften and protect the surface and to help application of make-up by providing a smooth base	Available for different skin types	After eye make-up removal, cleansing and toning and before make-up application – it is best applied about 10 minutes before make-up	Apply with fingers and hands, following strokes used for the cleansing routine.

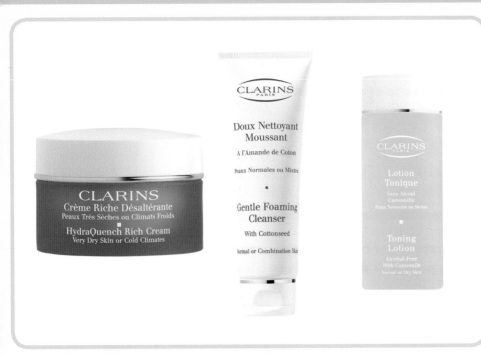

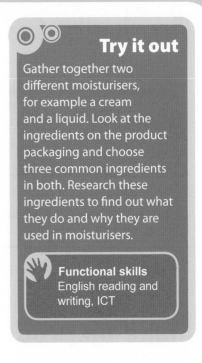

Try it out

Gather together two different moisturisers, for example a cream and a liquid. Look at the ingredients on the product packaging and choose three common ingredients in both. Research these ingredients to find out what they do and why they are used in moisturisers.

Functional skills
English reading and writing, ICT

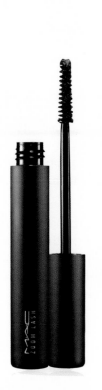

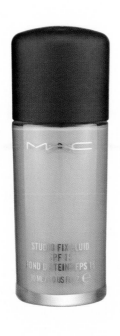

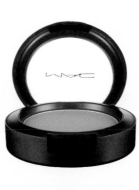

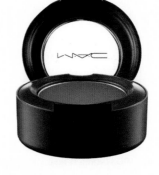

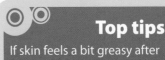

Top tips

If skin feels a bit greasy after putting on moisturiser, just blot the extra from the skin with a split tissue.

Use make-up that hasn't been tested on animals and is kind to the environment.

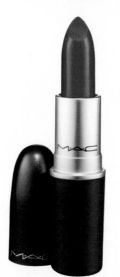

You should carry out a full cleanse using appropriate products before applying make-up

Just checking

1 When should you apply a toner?

2 How long should you wait after moisturising before applying make-up?

Products for make-up (2)

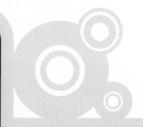

Q Many make-up artists swear by a favourite product. What is your favourite make-up product? What can't you do without and why?

Make-up products

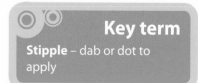

Key term

Stipple – dab or dot to apply

Product	Purpose	Information	When to use	How to use
Concealer	To cover up spots, blemishes and dark circles	Comes in a tube, jar or stick	Can be applied before or after foundation	Scrape a small amount onto a spatula with a brush, then **stipple** using a clean fingertip, blending gradually until the spot or blemish is covered.
Foundation	To provide a smooth, even base to the skin	It should be as close to natural skin tone as possible. It comes in a tube or jar, and can be cream/oil based, mousse or all-in-one, which means it is a foundation and powder together	Before or after concealer	Use a make-up sponge to apply foundation in smooth downward strokes, taking care not to apply to hairline or eyebrows. Blend it well and fade out at the jawline.
Powder	Sets the foundation and makes it last longer	Powder can come in a compact or loose. It is also available in a range of skin tone colours	After foundation and concealer	Apply using a cotton wool ball and/or powder brush.
Eyeshadow	To add colour and shape to the eyes	Comes in cream or powder and in a variety of colours. Some are matt while others are shimmery	After foundation, powder and concealer	Apply using a clean shadow applicator, using an eyeshadow brush to blend after applying the colour.

Eyeliner/eye pencil	Adds shape and depth to the eyes, making them look larger or wider	Comes in liquid, pencil, cake or pen applicator	Apply after eyeshadow but before mascara	Use a disposable eyeliner brush where possible or if using a pencil, sharpen it between clients. Pen applicators are not hygienic for use on clients as you cannot use a brush with them so only use them for yourself. Apply gently with a steady hand.
Mascara	Makes the lashes look fuller and longer	Some mascara is waterproof. There are a range of different shaped brushes in mascaras for different purposes, for example, lengthening and separating	After eyeshadow and eyeliner	Dip a clean disposable mascara brush into the mascara and use to apply to the eyelashes. Apply downwards on the top lashes first and then ask the client to look up so that you can coat the underneath of the top lashes. Then apply to the bottom lashes. Allow each coat to dry before applying another coat.
Blusher	Used to give colour and warmth to the cheeks and give the face shape	Comes in cream or powder	Powder blusher – apply after foundation and powder Cream blusher – after foundation but before powder	Powder – apply using a clean blusher brush, building up colour gradually. Cream – apply using a make-up sponge.
Lip liner	Used to improve the shape of the lips and to stop the lipstick spreading out	Comes in a range of different colours to match skin tone and lipstick colour	Use before applying lipstick	With a steady hand apply lip liner pencil to the outside edge of the lips. Don't press hard – apply using light feathery strokes.
Lipstick	Adds colour and texture to the whole face as well as to the lips. It finishes off the whole make-up.	Comes in many colours and textures	Use after lip liner pencil	Use a clean lip brush to apply colour to the lips.
Lip gloss	Adds shine to the lipstick or can be used on its own without lipstick	Comes in many colours	Use instead of lipstick or on top of	Use a clean lip brush to apply gloss to the lips.

Just checking

1 What make-up product is used to cover up spots and blemishes?

2 What should you use to apply foundation?

Try it out

- Research the make-up companies that test their products on animals and those that don't. Create a table or graph to show your results.

Functional skills
English reading and writing, ICT internet research, Mathematics graphs and charts

Factors influencing make-up (1)

Q When you look around you, which is the most common face shape you can see? Which do you think looks the most attractive?

Face shape

A person's face shape can influence the make-up techniques and colours you use. The same make-up can look very different on different face shapes. For example, what looks good on an oval shape may not be the most flattering for a square, oblong or round face shape. If you experiment with different colours and make-up application techniques, it will help you to understand how make-up can completely change a person's look.

Round	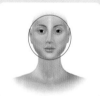	A round face has full cheeks and is usually quite short in length.
Oval	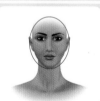	This is thought to be the ideal face shape.
Square	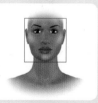	The forehead and jawline is quite straight.
Oblong	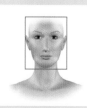	This face shape can be quite long and sometimes thin.

Try it out

It is not always easy to decide which face shape a person has. Practise this with friends. Pull your hair back in a ponytail and remove earrings and jewellery around the neck. Look carefully at each other and discuss which face shape you think you all are.

✋ **Functional skills**
English speaking

Skin type

There are four main skin types:

- Normal – this is most common in children and teenagers. It is clear, supple and smooth.
- Dry – this will feel very dry to touch. The skin does not shine and can feel tight due to lack of oil.
- Oily – this skin type will look shiny and feel greasy and can have spots and blackheads.
- Combination – normal or dry but with an oily T-section down the middle from the forehead down the nose to the chin. It will look shiny on the oily part.

For more information on the structure and function of the skin, look back to *Anatomy and physiology*, pages 70–71.

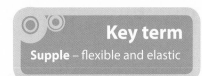
Key term

Supple – flexible and elastic

How skin type and texture can affect make-up

Skin type and texture can affect the application of make-up. They can also affect how long the make-up will last on the skin. For example:

- Dry or flaky skin can prevent the make-up from going on smoothly. It will also need a richer moisturiser underneath the make-up base.
- If a client has oily skin the make-up may not last as long. This is because the oily surface can cause the make-up to rub or slide off easily.
- If a client has skin with lots of spots or blemishes, or if it is uneven in colour and texture, a foundation base with good coverage is needed. Whereas, a clear, smooth and normal skin type could have a light cover of foundation and powder.

Eye, hair and skin colour

Although eyeshadow colours do not need to be the same colour as a person's eyes, you will find that some colours just don't look right. This is more to do with the natural tone of the person's skin, hair and eyes as a whole rather than one thing.

Some skin and hair has warm tones while others have cool tones. It is this, combined with eye colour, that will determine whether certain make-up colours look right. Warm make-up colours such as browns, creams and rusty colours may not look right on a person with very dark hair, pale skin and blue eyes.

In your class group there will be a range of different eye, hair and skin colours. Experiment on each other with different make-up colours.

Top tip

Remember that if the client wears glasses this can alter the appearance of the eye make-up. This will depend on whether the lenses in the glasses make the eyes appear smaller or larger.

Just checking

1 What sort of moisturiser should you use before make-up application for a dry skin type?

2 List the four basic face shapes.

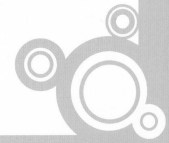

Factors influencing make-up (2)

Think of different make-up styles and trends. How have these been influenced by cultural influences?

Occasion

The type of make-up depends on what the client is doing. For example:

- Bridal and wedding make-up should be natural looking and long lasting. It also needs to look good in daylight. Usually the client will want the make-up to complement her outfit and flowers.
- Work – this type of make-up should be practical, long lasting and fairly natural. Shocking colours and techniques would not be suitable for most places of work.
- Evening out – whether it's a party, nightclub or meal in a restaurant, most people like to make the extra effort with clothing and make-up. It is acceptable to use more make-up, brighter colours and more daring application techniques (such as liquid eyeliners, red lipsticks and glittery eyeshadows).

Fashion trends

Make-up products, colours and techniques change often with the latest fashions. But most make-up and fashion trends come and go. In the 1960s liquid eyeliner and false eyelashes were in fashion and are popular again now. Celebrities and the media also influence make-up trends.

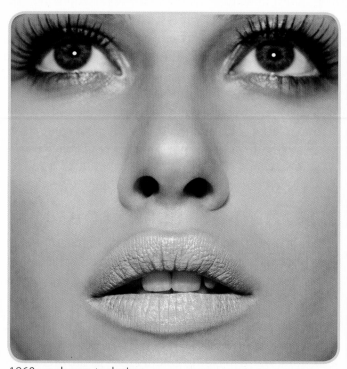

1960s make-up techniques

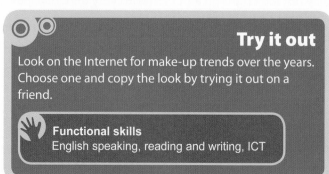

Try it out

Look on the Internet for make-up trends over the years. Choose one and copy the look by trying it out on a friend.

Functional skills
English speaking, reading and writing, ICT

Cultural factors

Countries, religions and beliefs can influence the make-up products and techniques used. But whoever and wherever you are, one of the easiest ways to improve your confidence is by applying make-up.

Over the years people have used all sorts of things to beautify their skin and appearance. Some were safe while others were not. The Romans and Egyptians used dangerous chemicals to stain their skin. Fortunately, things have improved but the desire to look good is still very important to us.

What may seem to you like an unusual way to make-up the skin is normal for someone else. It is important that we respect those differences.

Top tip

Look at magazines, television and other media to get ideas for different types of make-up for different occasions.

Lighting

If the lighting is wrong the effect of the make-up can be lost. If possible, make-up should be applied using the same light that the finished result will be shown in.

The following lighting is the most common:

- Daylight – the clearest but also the most **revealing**. In this lighting, blue is the main colour to show through.
  Occasion – bridal make-up

- Electric light bulb – this has a warm yellow glow. Purple colours may look greyish under this light and reds can lose some of their shade. This is even more extreme in candle light.
  Occasion – dinner party at home

- Fluorescent light – this produces a blue background colour which makes colours look cold. Most colours under this light look weaker, and orange looks greyish. However, blues look more **intense**.
  Occasion – nightclub

- Spotlight – this usually has a blue/white colour. Reddish colours, look deeper and the make-up overall should be clear and definite as everything can appear pale.
  Occasion – stage/theatre make-up

- Halogen – this is a very harsh white light that has a bleaching effect on all colours. It is essential to **emphasise** the make-up more so that it doesn't seem to disappear.
  Occasion – studio lighting for photo shoot

Key terms

Revealing – shows everything up
Intense – deeper and more powerful
Emphasise – make stronger

Just checking

1   What sort of make-up would be suitable for weddings?

2   How does fluorescent light affect make-up appearance?

3   What fashion trends were popular in the 1960s?

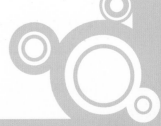

Prepare for make-up

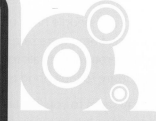

In this topic you will learn about:

- Preparing yourself, your client and your work area for make-up
- Following safe and hygienic working practices
- Communicating and acting in a professional manner

Q All make-up products must be safe for use on the skin. What legal authority in the UK is responsible for making sure make-up is safe to use?

Preparing yourself and your work area

The tools, equipment and products that you will need were covered on pages 178–83. You now need to lay these out on your trolley so that they are easy to reach. Before using your tools and equipment they should be cleaned and sterilised.

Top tip

Lay out your brushes and make-up products in the order that they need to be used. This will help to remind you of each stage.

Safe and hygienic working practices

Health, safety and hygiene always come first. They are covered in detail in *Follow health and safety in the salon*. Never forget how easy it is to cross-infect. Make sure that you use hygienic working practices at all times during your make-up treatment.

Brushes and make-up sponges, especially when damp, will encourage bacterial growth. It is essential that they are washed, air dried and stored in a dry area to reduce harmful bacteria.

Communication and behaviour

Always remember to behave appropriately and communicate in a positive way with your clients and colleagues. More information on this can be found in *Presenting a professional image in a salon*.

Preparing your client

Consultation

Welcome your client and introduce yourself so that they feel at ease and start to feel confidence in you. Ask them to take a seat while you go through a few questions for your records.

You will need to use a record card to write down important information during the consultation with your client.

The consultation process should cover the following:
- Personal client contact details
- Contra-indications or disorders of the skin and/or eyes
- Skin condition and skin type
- Make-up products and techniques used
- Your name
- Date of treatment
- Client signature

Certain conditions of the skin and general health may influence whether you can continue with a treatment. You may need to stop the treatment or alter it to suit the client and their skin type.

Carry out a visual study (see below) of the skin before you start.

Visual study of the skin

After you have filled in the record card, look carefully at the client's face shape, skin tone and texture. To see the client's face shape properly, push their hair away from their face with a headband. Also look at their eye and hair colour. All this information will help you to choose the most suitable make-up products and colours.

Most importantly, look for any contra-indications that may prevent or restrict treatment. If you think that a client has a contra-indication, check with your tutor before going ahead with the treatment. It is not up to you to decide if it is safe to carry on.

Client comfort

When you have completed the visual study, position the client on a make-up chair or couch. Make sure they are comfortable.

Use a gown or towel across the client's chest area or a make-up cape, to protect her clothing.

If the client needs head and neck support, give them a pillow or neck cushion.

Make sure that the lighting is not too bright and that the room is warm but not too stuffy. The atmosphere should be calm.

Ask the client to remove any jewellery and place it in their bag (then you won't be responsible if it goes missing).

Just checking

1 What should you look for when carrying out a visual study of the skin before make-up?

2 State four things that will need to be recorded on a client record card for make-up.

3 How do you make sure that sponges and brushes are clean and hygienic?

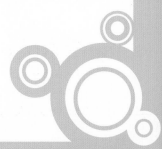

Applying basic make-up

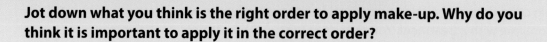

In this topic you will learn about:

- Applying basic make-up under supervision

Q Jot down what you think is the right order to apply make-up. Why do you think it is important to apply it in the correct order?

You are going to cover the stages required to carry out a basic make-up. It is important to think about the colours and techniques that will improve the client's natural good features and appearance. Following these simple steps will help you to develop more advanced techniques in the future. These could include those used for television, theatre and special occasions.

Try it out

Create a sheet that can be used to record the colours you use for each make-up. Make it visual, for example, lots of boxes or a face where make-up can be smudged on with clear labels to write the colours used. This would be very useful so that you could do the same make-up again.

Functional skills
English reading and writing, ICT

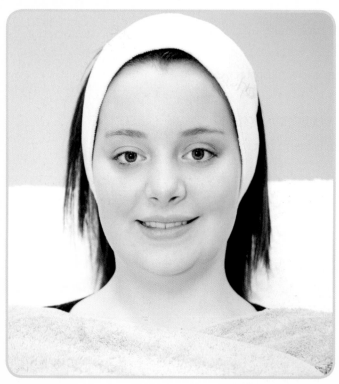

Before make-up

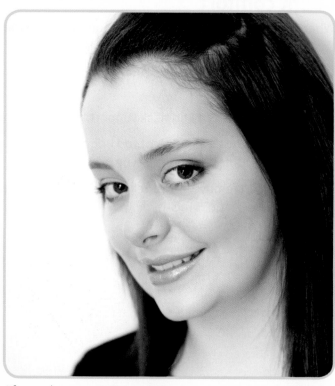

After make-up

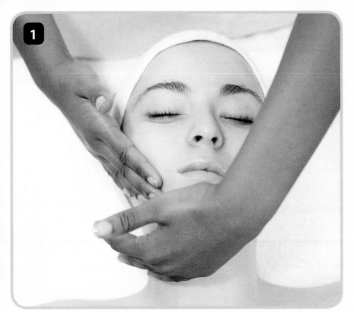

1

Follow the cleansing routine movements on page 150 of *Skin care* to complete the cleansing, toning and moisturising stages. These steps must be completed to make sure that the skin is very clean before you apply make-up

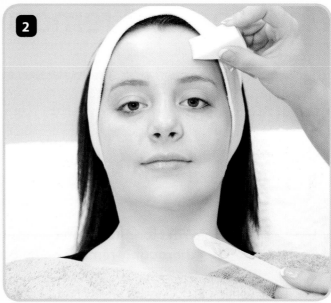

2

Apply foundation with a latex make-up sponge in downwards movements, taking care that you avoid the hairline and eyebrows. This will make sure that you don't get foundation in the hair or make it look thick and blotchy.

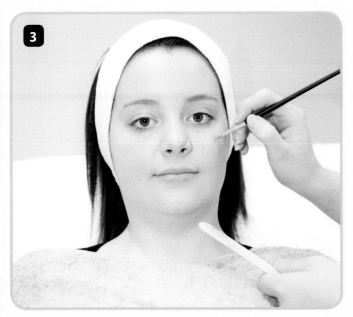

3

Apply concealer with a small brush and stipple it with a clean finger to blend it in.

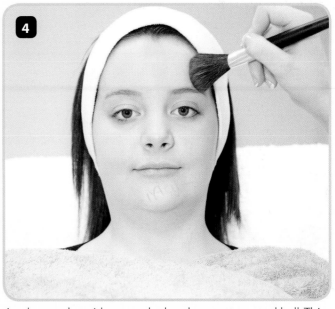

4

Apply powder with a powder brush or cotton wool ball. This is to set the foundation and concealer and stop the skin looking shiny.

Just checking

1 What is the purpose of lip liner?

2 What is the purpose of powder?

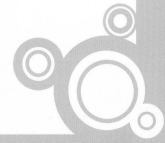

Top tip

The first stages are the most important for providing a smooth complexion, so don't rush the foundation, concealer and powder application.

Applying and removing basic make-up

In this topic you will learn about:

- Applying basic make-up under supervision
- Removing basic make-up under supervision

Q **What long-term effects could skin suffer from if you don't thoroughly remove make-up properly?**

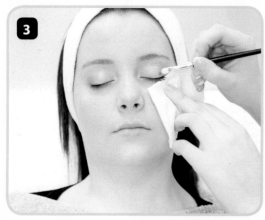

Apply blusher a little at a time by using a blusher brush. This will prevent you from applying too much colour at once.

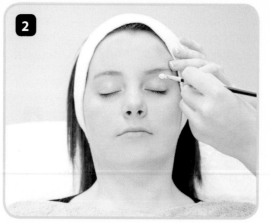

Apply eyeshadow using the sponge applicator. Blend colours well to avoid hard lines. The soft eye brush is good for blending once colour has been applied. Use the lightest colour underneath the brow bone, adding darker colours to the lid.

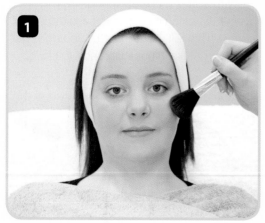

Apply darker colours to the eyelid and blend well, using a tissue to protect smudging of colours under the eye.

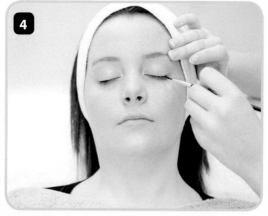

Apply eyeliner with an eyeliner brush or use eye pencil. Apply as close to the lashes as you can. If it is too dark you can soften it by applying eye shadow over the top or smudging it with a clean cotton bud. Eyeliner and pencil give depth to the eyes.

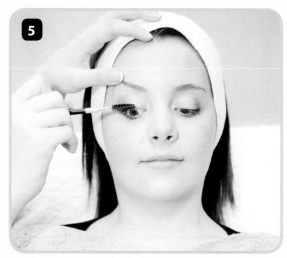

Apply mascara to the lashes using even, light strokes. Use an eyelash comb to separate the hairs. Mascara will complete the finished look and make the eyes appear bigger.

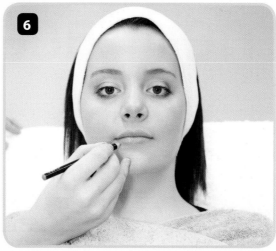

Gently apply the lip liner on the outside edge of the lips. To steady your hand you may find it easy to balance your hand on the client's chin. Lip liner helps the lipstick stay on better and also helps to correct any uneven lips.

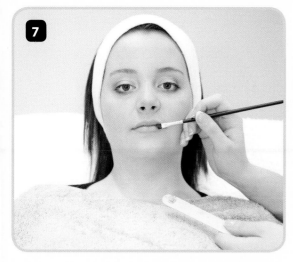

Apply lipstick with a clean lip brush. Lipstick will balance the rest of the make-up, adding colour and interest. Apply a lip gloss that is clear or complements the lipstick colour using a clean lip brush. Lip gloss will add shine and complete the whole make-up look.

Make-up removal

Your client will need to know how to remove her make-up thoroughly and safely. Advise her how to:

1   massage eye make-up remover gently around the eye area, taking care not to get it in the eyes

2   use a clean ball of cotton wool (damp or dry) to remove the make-up and eye make-up remover

3   cleanse, tone and moisturise the skin with gentle, smooth movements to make sure all the make-up is removed thoroughly.

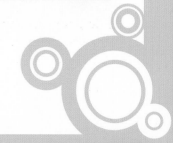

Top tips
Aftercare advice:

- Tell the client to make sure the make-up is removed thoroughly before going to bed.
- Don't touch the face as the make-up won't last as long.
- Tell the client to visit her GP if her skin becomes red or itchy as she may have an allergy to one of the products.

Just checking

1   Which brush is the best one for applying eyeshadow?

2   State three aftercare points that you would give to the client.

Themed face painting

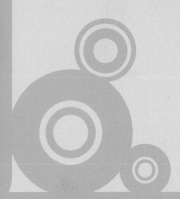

In this unit you will learn about:

- Products, tools and equipment for themed face painting
- Preparation of yourself, your client and your work area for themed face painting
- Factors that could influence themed face painting techniques
- Designing 2D images and adapting them to a 3D surface
- Applying and removing face painting

Introduction

When we think about face painting we tend to picture colourful designs painted onto children's faces at fairs and fêtes. In fact, face painting dates back thousands of years across many different cultures. It has been used for many purposes – and not just for fun. The history of face painting includes painting for religious and tribal purposes, camouflage and advertising, etc.

Themed face painting uses many different colours and techniques. All of these change the appearance of the face to create an **illusion**. In this unit you will learn how the art of themed face painting can be mastered with lots of practice. You should have lots of fun creating images such as animals, historical figures, flowers and masks using paint, glitter and stickers.

Top tips

- Check for allergies before you start.
- Make sure you have a good supply of fresh water for washing brushes and sponges throughout your painting.
- Allow colours to dry before adding second coats. The colour will be deeper and cleaner.
- Apply base colour with a damp sponge. Make sure it's not too wet otherwise you will get a streaky finish.
- Keep brush strokes even with a steady hand.

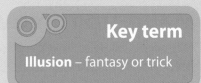

Key term

Illusion – fantasy or trick

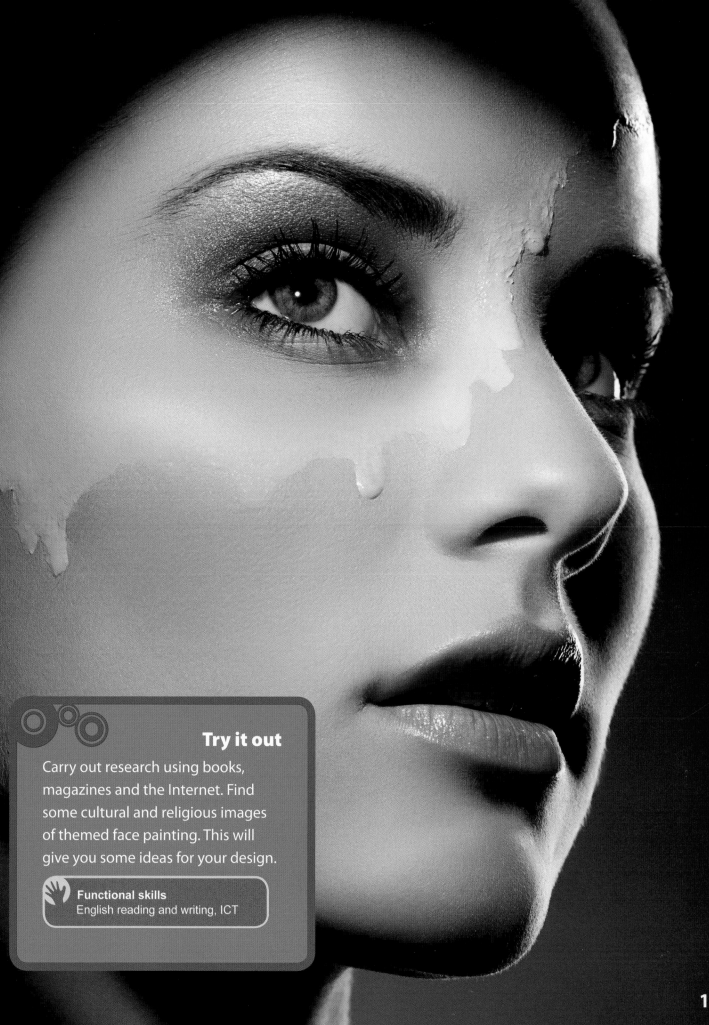

Try it out

Carry out research using books, magazines and the Internet. Find some cultural and religious images of themed face painting. This will give you some ideas for your design.

Functional skills
English reading and writing, ICT

Face painting products

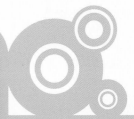

In this topic you will learn about:

- Products for themed face painting

Q Products, tools and equipment for face painting are quite easy to get hold of. Where do you think you could buy face paints, sponges, stencils and brushes?

To be able to carry out themed face painting you must first know how to set up your work area with the correct tools, products and equipment.

Brushes, stickers, sponges and a kaleidoscope of colours will help you to create fantastic images.

Products

Product	Purpose	Information	When to use	How to use
Eye make-up remover	To clean off eye make-up	Available as an oil, lotion or gel. Some remove waterproof make-up	Before make-up application	Use damp cotton wool squares and/or cotton buds to gently clean around the eyes and the eyelashes.
Cleansers	Used to remove make-up on the face and to clean dirt, dust and grime from the skin and pores.	Available in different types for different skins. See Skin care, page 146	After eye make-up removal	Use damp cotton wool squares and follow the cleansing routine from Skin care, page 152.
Cleansing wipes	Wipes that have cleansing products already on them	Easy to use and come in different strengths for different skin types	For removing face painting products from the skin or before face painting, to clean the skin	Wipe gently across the skin, taking care not to drag.
Soap or hand wash	To clean the hands before working on clients	Available as a block of soap or in a gel form that needs no water	This should be available to wash make-up off the hands and to clean the sponges	Soap – use with water. Gel – use a small amount to rub into your hands.
Toners	Used to remove any leftover cleanser from the skin. They also dissolve oil, refresh and cool the skin and tighten the pores	Available in different types for different skins	After cleansing and before moisturiser	Apply with damp cotton wool squares, following the same routine used to clean the face.

Moisturiser	Applied to the skin to soften it	Available for different skin types	After eye make-up removal, cleansing and toning and before make-up application. IMPORTANT Unless it is very dry it may be better to avoid using moisturiser as it could make the skin slightly oily. This means that the water-based face paints may go on very well but they could also smudge too easily.	Apply with fingers and hands, following the strokes used for the cleansing routine.

Non-toxic water-based face paints

These are safe and easy to use and can be washed off easily with water. They are also **hypo-allergenic** and **non-toxic**. They are applied with either a damp sponge or a brush and come in many different colours and types. For example, there are **metallic**, glitter or sparkle ones as well as just the plain coloured paints. They come in tubes, pots or as refills.

Glitters

Glitter for themed face painting can be loose. However, there is less chance of spillage if glitter gels are used. These come in tubes and can be applied with a small brush – there is a variety of colours. If you apply just a little to the design it can make a big difference to the finished result.

Stickers/transfers/ temporary tattoos and gems

These items are easy to peel and stick on. They are not permanent and don't need any glue to fix them to the skin. Therefore they are less likely to cause an allergy. Many designs are available such as diamonds, stars, flowers, people and patterns.

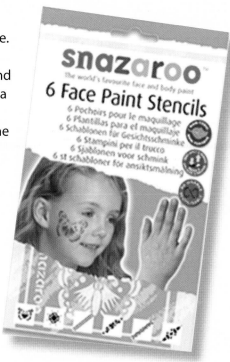

A stencil pack

Key terms

Hypo-allergenic – unlikely to cause an allergic reaction
Non-toxic – not poisonous
Metallic – shiny

Try it out

Find out the dates of local fêtes and carnivals. Ask if there will be face painting. See if you can spend a day watching so that you can pick up lots of helpful hints and tips.

Functional skills
English reading, speaking and listening

Top tip

Plan your design carefully. Choose colours and techniques that look good together to create a great face painting design.

Just checking

1 What are the two types of glitter?
2 Why should face paints be non-toxic and water-based?

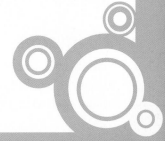

Tools and equipment for face painting

In this topic you will learn about:
- Tools and equipment for themed face painting

Q **Can you make a list of the different places and situations where you might carry out face painting techniques?**

Equipment

Mirror and lighting

A mirror and good lighting are very important for successful face painting. Lighting should be bright but must not cast shadows onto the face. Natural daylight is the best. A mirror should be available for checking the finished result.

Headbands

It is very important to make sure that the hair is off the face. It could be irritating to the person being made up and it will also affect the application of the make-up and smudge the colour. If you don't have a headband, use butterfly clips instead.

Gowns

Face painting can be messy so you must protect both your clothing and the model's. Gowns are best although old shirts or towels can also be used.

Towels

These are useful for different purposes. For example, a towel may be laid across the client's chest to protect their clothing if there is not a gown or make-up cape available.

Cotton wool

A selection of damp and dry cotton wool is useful for wiping and cleaning make-up palettes and brushes. It will also be useful when cleansing the skin and painting it.

2D images

Find images, photos or other pictures of animals, characters, superheroes or fantasy shapes to give you some ideas. You then need to adapt them to a 3D image such as onto a face, mask or mannequin.

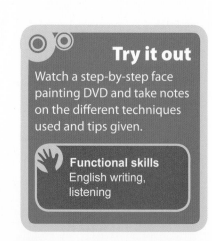

Try it out

Watch a step-by-step face painting DVD and take notes on the different techniques used and tips given.

Functional skills
English writing, listening

Tissues

Tissues are usually split in two as this is more economical and they also mould to the skin better. They are used to blot extra toner or moisturiser from the skin.

Bowls

Small plastic or metal bowls are needed to hold cotton wool and tissues.

Tools

Brushes

You will need different brushes for each stage of the make-up application. Thinner ones will be used for fine detail such as wisps and whiskers. Thicker brushes will be used to apply colour in large sections. A good set of brushes that is well looked after and cleaned properly will last you a long time.
The most important brushes to have are:

- fine flat face painting brush
- fine round face painting brush
- large flat face painting brush
- medium flat face painting brush
- medium round multi-purpose painting brush.

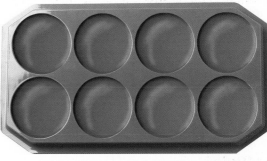

A face painting brush

Palette

This will be used to mix the water-based face paints to create new colours. You can also use it to deepen or soften existing colours. Because they are water paints, a traditional flat make-up palette will not be any good as the colours will run off. A palette with scooped circles is best if possible – if not, use a small bowl.

Face paints palette

Sponges

You will need two types of sponges:

- Latex sponge – these are high-density face painting sponges. This means that they have very small pores or holes in them and are good for covering areas with colour.
- Stipple sponge – this is a coarser sponge and can create different effects such as an unshaven look on a pirate, or facial hair.

Make-up case

Although not essential, this is very useful. Use it to keep all your tools, products and equipment together in one place.

Top tip

A great way to store all of your tools, products and equipment for face painting is in a box that pulls out and has lots of compartments. These are sometimes called fishing tackle boxes – of course use a new one!

Just checking

1 List three types of brushes that are used for face painting.

2 What types of sponges are used for face painting?

Factors influencing themed face painting

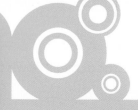

In this topic you will learn about:

- Factors that could influence themed face painting

How do you think you could become a face and body painter? What qualifications and training do you think you would need?

Size and shape of face

The size and shape of a person's face can influence the face painting techniques and amount of face paint you use. For example, if you are creating a design on a child their face is probably quite small. Therefore, you need to choose a design that will fit well onto the area of the face. More information on face shapes and how these can affect the look of a make-up is covered fully in *Basic make-up application*, pages 184–85.

Skin colour and type

Colours will need to be chosen carefully for the colour of the skin you are painting your design on. Darker skins will need colours that cover much better and are stronger and deeper than those used on a lighter skin. Water-based face paint covers well on most skin types.

However, if the skin is very oily, it is important to carry out a thorough cleanse first. If the skin is very dry and flaky, a small amount of moisturiser will help. But be careful not to use too much or the make-up will not last as long and it might even slide off.

Theme or occasion

The colours, techniques and products used will depend on the topical theme or occasion. For example, the make-up will be bright and colourful for a carnival theme. If you have chosen a Halloween theme, then the colours will probably be greens, blacks and oranges and the techniques used should create a scary look.

Age of client

Younger clients will probably enjoy being painted as cartoon characters and animals. Older clients (for example, teenagers) will prefer fantasy figures and masks with the use of glitters, transfers and gems.

Timings

The time you have available is important. Some designs are very **intricate** and need much more time than others. Think about this and choose a design that you have enough time to create.

Costing

A design that takes a lot of time is likely to cost more to do. Using lots of different colours and techniques (applying glitter, gems and transfers) will also cost more than a straightforward water-based face painting design. For example, if you are creating a design for someone visiting a carnival, your costs should be set according to the design chosen by the client.

Equipment needed and available

Pages 196–99 list most of the tools, products and equipment that you will need to complete lots of different designs. However, you may not have all of these. Be practical and work with what you do have to complete a design that is possible.

Adverse skin conditions and allergies

Skin conditions and allergies will influence whether you are able to create a themed face painting on someone's face. However, it is possible to work on a mannequin or face mask.

Gender and cultural factors

Different countries, religions, beliefs and gender can influence themed face painting designs, products and techniques. For example, at the Notting Hill Carnival (which is held every year in London) the theme is Caribbean.

Themed face painting on children at a village fête may mean that the boys choose action figure and cartoon character designs whereas girls may choose fairytale. This won't always be the case though, so always be aware of different people's **preferences**.

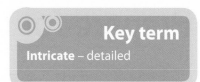

Key term

Intricate – detailed

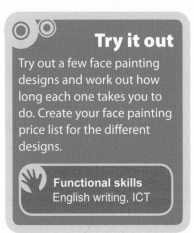

Try it out

Try out a few face painting designs and work out how long each one takes you to do. Create your face painting price list for the different designs.

Functional skills
English writing, ICT

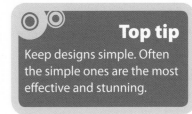

Key term

Preferences – choices

Just checking

1. Name three factors that influence themed face painting.
2. What are the typical designs that a young child might ask for?

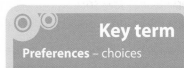

Top tip

Keep designs simple. Often the simple ones are the most effective and stunning.

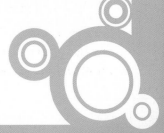

Prepare for themed face painting

In this topic you will learn about:

- Preparation of yourself, your client and your work area for themed face painting
- Communicating and acting in a professional manner
- Following safe and hygienic working practices

Apart from children, who else do you think may have themed face painting done? Make a list.

Setting up your work area

The tools, equipment and products that you will need were covered on pages 196–99. You now need to lay these out so that they are easy to reach. This may be on a trolley, a table or even a chair if you are at a carnival or fête. Make sure that you have covered the surface before setting out the make-up. Before using your tools and equipment they should be cleaned and sterilised.

Client preparation

Welcome the client or model and introduce yourself. Ask them to take a seat while you go through a few questions for your records. This can be difficult in a carnival or fête setting but you must ask people if they are allergic or sensitive to any make-up products or face painting.

Always be courteous and polite to the client. If you are doing face painting on small children, it is essential that you behave well, are patient and set a good example to them.

Further information on communication and behaviour can be found in *Presenting a professional image in a salon*.

Visual inspection

Before starting any face painting, chat to the client and ask if they have any problems with their skin or if they are allergic to any products. While you are doing this, look at the skin to see if there is anything that may prevent you from being able to apply the make-up.

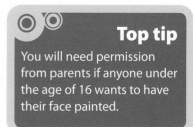

Top tip

You will need permission from parents if anyone under the age of 16 wants to have their face painted.

Client comfort

When you have completed the visual study, position the client on a chair, making sure they are comfortable.

Use a gown or towel across the chest area, or use a make-up cape, to protect the client's clothing. Cover the hair with a headband or clip it up away from the face.

Safe and hygienic working practices

Although health, safety and hygiene is covered in detail in *Follow health and safety in the salon*, never forget how easy it is to cross-infect. Make sure that you use hygienic working practices during your themed make-up. Brushes and make-up sponges, especially when damp, will encourage bacterial growth. They must be washed, air dried and stored in a dry area to reduce harmful bacteria. This must be done after every make-up. If you are going to do a lot of face painting, it is best to have plenty of make-up sponges as well as clean water and soap.

Try it out

Create a DIY face painting poster. Photograph each step as you do it so that you have a selection of step-by-step photographs to stick onto a large piece of card. Add a small description of what you have done for each stage – these are called captions.

Functional skills
English reading and writing, ICT

In the salon

Lian and her friend Lucy were very excited. They were going to run a children's face painting stall at their local carnival. Their tutor was going to meet them there with the **consent forms** for parents to sign. They were all prepared and ready to go and the children had already started queuing. It was a bit early, and their tutor hadn't arrived yet, but the girls decided to start. Lian did a lion design on the first little girl and she was delighted with it.

Lucy and Lian continued face painting the other children until they heard a loud shriek and saw a woman running towards them. She was the mother of the child with the lion design and she was furious. She said that her daughter suffered from allergies and was now itching and scratching. She shouted at them that they should not have painted her face without checking with her first.

- What should Lian and Lucy have done before applying face paint to the children? Why should they have waited for their tutor?

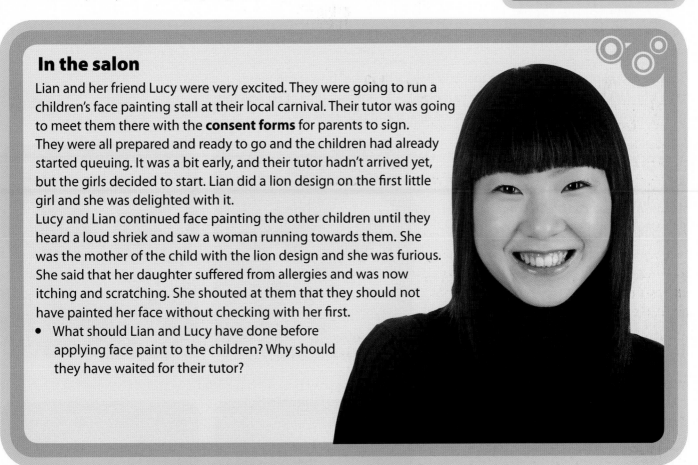

Just checking

1 How should you behave if you are carrying out face painting on a child?

2 What should you do before carrying out face painting on a child under 16?

Key term

Consent forms – permission forms allowing a person/child to have their face painted

Design a 3D image from a 2D image

Did you know that face and body art images have been created and used on billboards, in music videos and in fashion? Can you find some iconic music or fashion images?

You are going to recreate a 2D image that you have designed onto a 3D surface, such as a face or mask.

Take photographs of each step so that you have a record of how to do things next time. It's always good to be able to look back at photographs of completed designs, especially if you decide to become a face and body painter.

Types of images

There is a wide range of different images that you can create. Here are just a few examples.

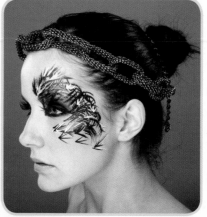

Fantasy

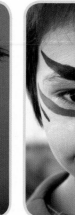

Cartoon fantasy figure

Designing your 2D image

You may decide to design your own 2D image completely but make sure you get lots of ideas first.

Explore designs from a range of places such as:

- comics and magazines
- Internet images that you can print off
- historical books
- science and nature books
- art and design images
- photographs.

Remember, the design you choose should reflect your personality and your skills.

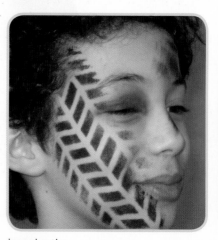

Imaginative

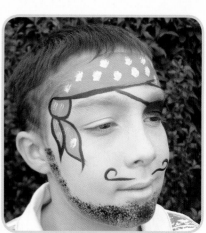

Pirate

Planning your design

Planning is important to the success of any themed face painting. Look at the image as a whole and then break it down into small easy steps that build up to the finished design.

The first thing you will always do is prepare the skin. Next you will cover the skin with a base colour so that you can paint your design onto it.

Practise with simple designs first. As you get more skilled you can try out different techniques. You must be able to complete your design in the time you have. You also need to bear in mind which tools, equipment and products are available.

Face painting techniques

Sponging

Use damp latex sponges. Cover them in water-based face paint and apply with smooth strokes to cover the face or surface. Over-stroking will result in streaks, so don't do this. Also, water-based face paint dries very quickly – work quickly to cover the area before the paint dries. Use fresh cold water to dampen the sponge again. You will also need water to rinse out one colour before using the sponge for the next one.

Painting

Load your brush with face paint and use steady even strokes to paint lines, whiskers, dots, etc. onto the face. Try to keep the painting **symmetrical**.

Stippling

Dip the brush into the required colour and use a pressing action to create a shadow or **mottled** effect, such as a beard.

Aftercare and removal of face paints

- Remove the water-based face paint colours using damp cotton wool with cleanser on it or use cleansing wipes.
- The glitter gel may need a thicker cleansing cream that you massage into the glitter and then wipe off.
- If you use soap and water to remove the face paint, make sure that you dry it well with a clean towel afterwards so that the client's skin doesn't get sore.

Just checking

1 How should you remove water-based face paints?

2 How should you remove glitter and glitter gels?

Key terms

Symmetrical – both sides are balanced
Mottled – patchy and spotty

Try it out

Visit www.pearsonhotlinks.co.uk for a list of face painting websites. Enter the express code P7511. Use these websites to research 2D images that you can re-create onto a 3D surface.

Functional skills
English reading, ICT

Top tip

Visit YouTube on the Internet and search 'face painting'. You will find some fun video clips showing you how to do different designs.

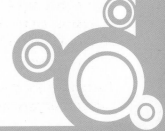

Carry out themed face painting techniques

Before you start, cleanse and tone the skin. If the skin is very dry you may need to also apply a small amount of moisturiser.

Step-by-step tiger

1

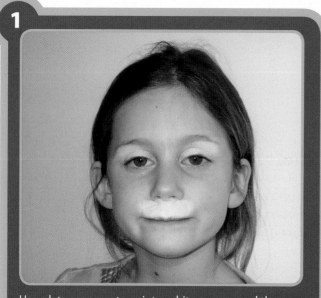

Use a latex sponge to paint a white area around the mouth and eyes.

2

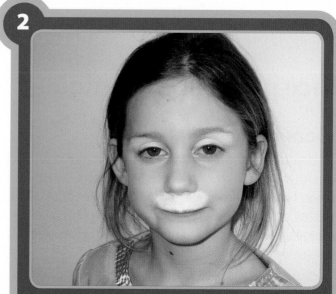

Use another clean sponge to apply yellow around the eyes, cheeks and chin.

3

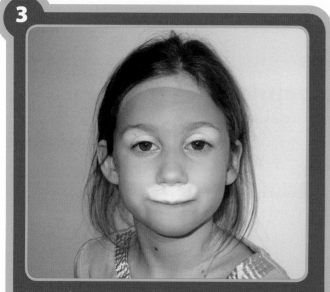

Use another sponge to add orange around the outside of the face. Blend the orange and yellow together by going slightly over the edges of the yellow paint with the orange. If the paint is too dark you can keep blending using the yellow and orange sponges until you get the effect you like.

4

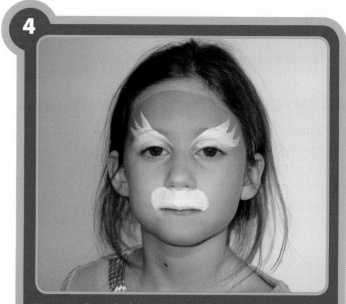

Use a medium thick brush to paint white eyebrows above the eyes. Use the line of the client's actual eyebrow as a guide, lifting the brush at the end of the stroke to create the point. It is sometimes easier to paint the side you feel least confident with first.

5

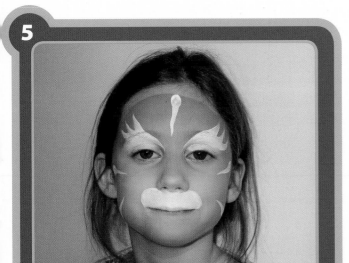

Add white stripes. Start your brush strokes at the outer edge of the orange paint and drag in. If you lift the brush as you drag, it will create a tapered look to the stripes. Still using the white paint, place a thin line under each eye.

6

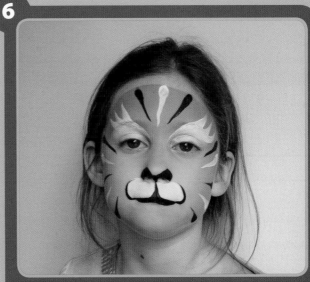

Use black paint to add a nose. Follow the natural flare of the nostrils to make sure both sides are even. Use the black to add a line from under the nose to the top lip. This should get larger as you go down to include the top lip. Paint both lips black. Add black stripes in the same way as the white stripes.

7

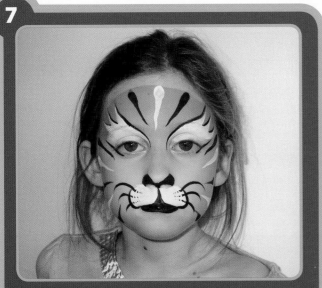

Add brush strokes around the mouth to create the whiskers. If you lift the brush at the end of the stroke and flick the tip you can achieve a pointed look. Use a thin brush to add small dots above the top lip and outline the whiskers and eyebrows for definition.

Nail art

Introduction

Nail decoration goes back centuries when ingredients such as gelatin, beeswax and colourings were first used to create nail paints. As science and technology improved, excellent quality nail varnishes were created in a fantastic range of colours and finishes.

Most recently nails have been decorated with accessories. These include stickers, gems, stencils and even real crystals, as well as creative painting techniques. These have all helped to make nail art a popular and beautiful addition to nails.

Top tip

Don't be afraid to experiment with your designs. There is no right or wrong way to be creative!

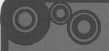

Try it out

Create a colourful wall chart or poster that shows the history of nail art. Use lots of images and clear labels to show how nail art has developed over the years.

Functional skills
English reading and writing

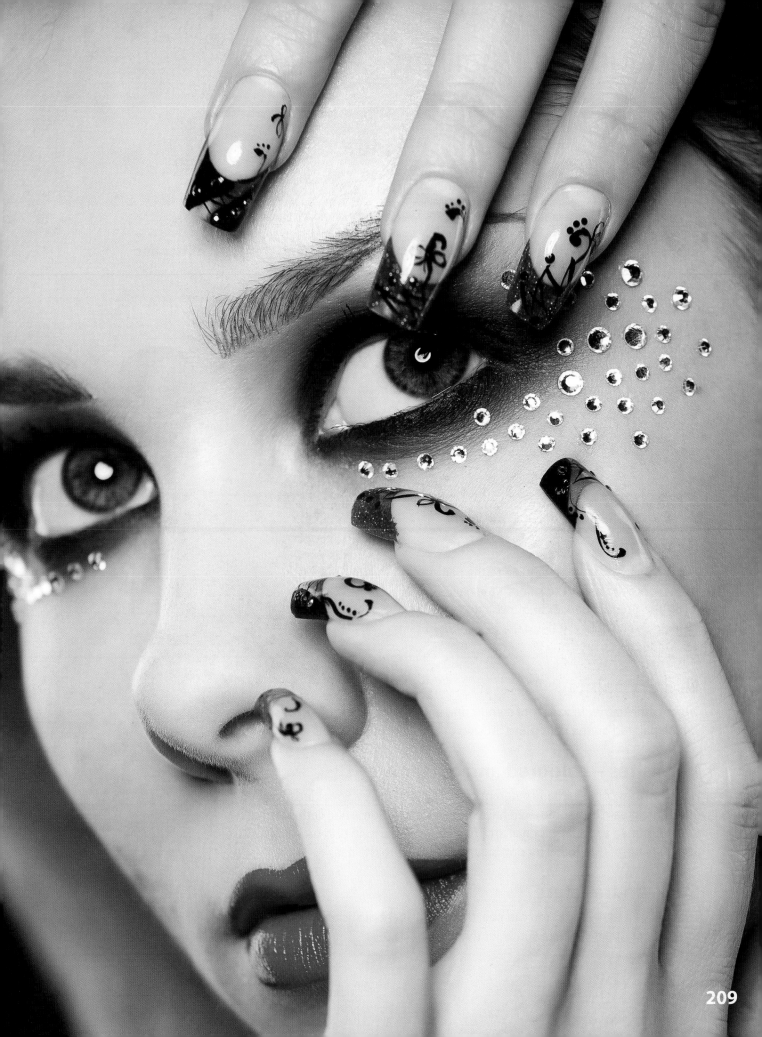

Products for nail art

In this topic you will learn about:

- Products for basic nail art techniques

Q **Nail art designs can be created with paint, transfers, glitter and stickers. How else can nails be decorated?**

Nail art is great fun and gives you a chance to express your creativity and imagination.

It's economical too because decorative items such as glitter, gemstones and transfers will last a long time. There will be enough in each pack to do lots of nails if you make sure you put lids back on to avoid spilling them.

Products

Base coat

This is usually clear and is applied to the nail plate before the nail art to smooth the nail. It will also prevent dark or bright colours staining the nail plate. It helps the design to last longer.

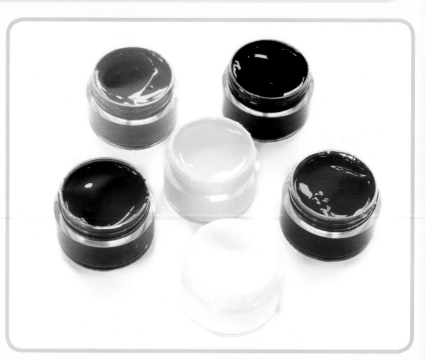

Nail art paints

Nail art paints

These come in a wide variety of colours and are usually water-based. Designs can be painted on the nails using brushes and special effects tools.

Varnishes – coloured and glitter

Nail varnishes come in many different colours and textures. Some are metallic, others are cream and some even have glitter in them. Some nail varnishes have been designed especially for nail art. They come with a long thin brush as well as a small piece of thin metal for dotting the varnish onto the nail.

Stick-on transfers

These have a sticky back. You can peel them off a sheet of stickers and attach to the place on the nail where you want them.

Top tip

When applying flat shapes, gemstones and chunky glitter to the nail, put a small piece of Blu-Tack® on the end of an orange wood stick. The gem or glitter will stick to the Blu-Tack so that you can put your decoration in the correct place on the nail. It will come off easily from the Blu-Tack as it doesn't stick too much.

Flat shapes

There are lots of bright colours and shapes to choose from. They are easy to apply as they stick to wet nail varnish.

Gemstones

These look like real precious stones. They come in lots of different colours and are easy to apply. They stick to wet varnish.

Foils, foil sealer and adhesive

Foils come in many different designs. You need to practise applying foils but the results can be stunning. Apply foil adhesive to the nail. Wait until it becomes clear and then put the foil onto the nail and press down. Gently rub it and then remove it carefully. The design will be on the nail. Then seal the design with foil sealer.

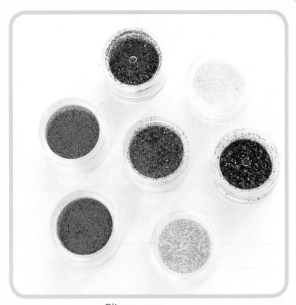

Glitter pots

Glitter

This will bring your nail art alive – whether you use a glitter varnish or loose glitter dust. The easiest way to apply glitter dust is to first coat the nail with base coat. To coat the tip only, dip the end of the nail into the glitter, or you can sprinkle it on the wet base coat all over the nail. You can also use chunky glitter (which is unusually shaped). Apply it using an orange wood stick.

Striping tape

This comes in many colours. It is on a roll and is made from a very thin foil that is self-adhesive. It measures about 1 mm thick and is used to create stripes on the nail.

Finishing sealer or top coat

This is a clear sealer that is used to seal the finished nail art design. This will prevent it from chipping and peeling, therefore making it last longer. It also adds a lovely shine to the finished design.

Non-acetone nail varnish remover

This nail varnish remover does not have acetone in it so it will not melt the artificial nail structure. It is also less drying to the natural nail.

Artificial nail structure

These are used to create your designs on. They can be fiddly to hold so it is best to mount them onto a piece of card or an upturned cardboard box. Fix them down with Blu-Tack and then start your design.

Top tips

If you are using water-based paints, clean your tools and brushes and correct any mistakes by wiping over with water. Do not use nail varnish remover.

Advise clients to apply a top coat over the design every other day to prevent the design chipping.

Try it out

Visit some companies on the Internet that supply tools, products and equipment. Work out how much it would cost you to set up a nail art kit with all the things that you need.

Functional skills
English reading and writing, Mathematics, ICT

Just checking

1 Why shouldn't you use nail varnish remover that contains acetone?

2 Name two types of glitter.

Tools and equipment for nail art

In this topic you will learn about:
- Tools and equipment for basic nail art techniques

Q What sort of nail art designs can be created with an airbrushing tool?

Tool or equipment	Use
Special effects tool (dotting tool) – two ends, one small ball and one large	Dip the small or large balled end into paint and create dots on the nail
Striping brush	Dip into paint and use slow movements to create stripes or zigzags or quick flicking movements to create flicks and wisps
Fine detailer brush	This is used to paint detail
Fan brush	These are used for striping and layering multiple colours onto your nails, different from the straight lines from striping brushes as the effect with a fan brush can be like an airbrushed effect

Nail files and emery boards

These are used to file down the artificial or natural nails or to smooth rough edges.

Orange wood sticks

These are used to attach gemstones, chunky glitter and flat shapes to the nail.

General purpose rounded safety scissors

These are used for cutting the striping tape, which your tutor will do for you.

Cotton buds

These are used for any cleaning up you need to do on or around the nail.

Card or small upturned cardboard box

This is used for mounting the artificial nail structures to make it easier to work on them.

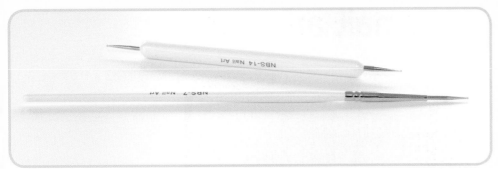

Dotting tools

Top tip

Blu-Tack can be attached to an orange wood stick to pick up gems, chunky glitter and flat shapes. They can then be put in place on the nail.

Try it out

Make a nail art design scrapbook.
Research some websites to find some 2D images that you can recreate onto a 3D surface. Print off some of the images. Add short descriptions next to the designs to say how they are done.

Functional skills
English reading and writing, ICT

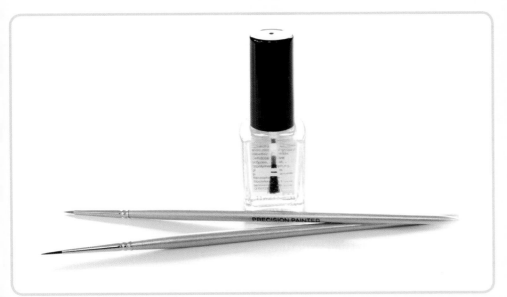

A selection of striping brushes and top coat

In the salon

Shabeena had bought lots of glitter, gemstones and flat shapes to add to her nail art collection. She couldn't wait to try out some new designs.

During her next lesson she laid out everything on her trolley and opened them up so they were easy to reach and use. Shabeena then realised she didn't have any water to rinse her brushes. She got up quickly and knocked over her new products. The glitter, tiny gemstones and shapes went all over the trolley and floor. Shabeena burst into tears.

- How could Shabeena have avoided this happening?

Just checking

1 What is the difference between the effects of a striping brush and a fan brush?

2 List three pieces of tools and equipment for nail art.

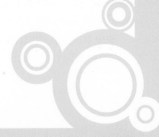

Factors influencing nail art design

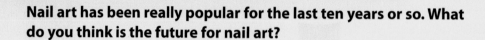

Q Nail art has been really popular for the last ten years or so. What do you think is the future for nail art?

The same nail art design would not be suitable for everyone. There are many things to consider so that you can create a design that suits the purpose, the lifestyle and the nails themselves. This section covers the different factors that may influence nail art design.

Length of nails

The nail art design applied to the natural nail, or an artificial nail structure, depends on the length. Very short nails will not allow much of a design to be created. They require very simple techniques that will fit on the space available.

Nail shape

The shape of the nails will affect the design chosen. Some designs look better on rounded or square shaped nails. Others look better on pointed nails, especially if the theme is something like Halloween.

Occasion

Nail art provides the finishing touch for any outfit, make-up or hairstyle. Designs should be chosen depending on the purpose. For example:
- a simple design with pale colours is suitable for work (perhaps a French manicure with transfers)
- funky bright colours and glitter with foil stripes are suitable for a night out or a fashion show.

Fashion trends

Nail techniques have always been influenced by fashion – nail art in particular. Celebrities and models often help to make nail art fashionable because we see them with the latest colours, designs and techniques on their own nails. A celebrity may also advertise them.

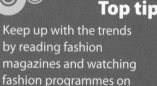

Top tip
Keep up with the trends by reading fashion magazines and watching fashion programmes on the television. You will get ideas to create your designs to complement the latest trends in clothes, hair and make-up.

Social and cultural factors

There are many cultures around the world. For some people, hand and nail decoration are part of their religious beliefs. In some eastern parts of the world people paint their hands and nails with Henna (which stains the fingernail and skin).

Also people now have more **disposable income** and are more aware of different treatments and services available to them.

Nail growth rate

If nail art is applied to the natural nail or onto acrylic nails, the design may need re-doing when the natural nail grows.

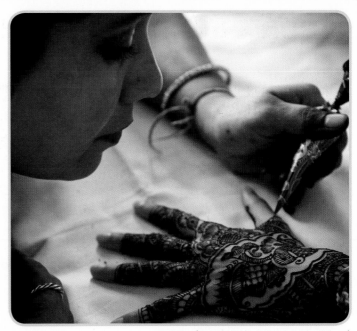

Using henna

Skin colour

Choose colours of paint and nail varnish that complement the client's skin tone on her hands. Skin has different underlying tones to it. For example:
- blue skin tone – avoid bright pink nail colours and go for more neutral colours
- yellow skin tone – these clients can sometimes be quite tanned so bright pinks, reds and greens will complement their skin tone.

Key term

Disposable income – the money available to spend when tax and bills have been taken out

Time available

Some designs can be very time-consuming and more complicated than others. Make sure that you have enough time to do the design you have chosen.

Pricing of treatment

The more time a design takes, the more it will cost in a salon. If the design uses more expensive products, this should also be considered when a salon is setting their prices.

Try it out

Visit some local salons and find out how much they charge for nail art designs. Also ask what sort of nail art they do. Display your findings on a graph to show the most popular designs and the most expensive designs.

Functional skills
English speaking, reading and writing, Mathematics

Adverse skin and nail conditions

Skin and nail conditions and allergies will influence whether you are able to create a nail art design on a person's natural nails or artificial/acrylic nails. However, if you are working on an artificial nail structure this won't matter.

Just checking

1 Name three factors that could influence nail art design.

2 What colours would be best for someone with blue tones to their skin?

Prepare for nail art design

How many nail infections could you get from using dirty tools?

Your work area should be well prepared, whatever treatment you are carrying out. This will help you gain the confidence of those around you including clients, colleagues and tutors. Sloppy working methods and untidy work areas can lead to accidents, cross-infection and poor techniques.

Setting up your work area

The tools, equipment and products that you need were covered on pages 210–13. You now need to lay these out so that they are easy to reach. Before using your tools and equipment they should be cleaned and sterilised.

Top tip

Make sure you spend time preparing, even though you will be keen to move on to the practical skills of designing your nail art. This will save you time later and will make you more organised.

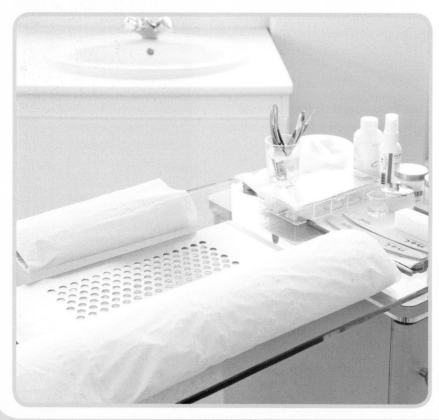

A nail work station

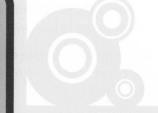

Safe and hygienic working practices

Although health, safety and hygiene is covered in detail in *Follow health and safety in the salon* you still need to think about how easy it is to cross-infect. Make sure that you use hygienic working practices during your nail art design. Brushes, especially when damp, will encourage bacterial growth. Therefore, they must be washed, air dried and stored in a dry area to reduce harmful bacteria. This must be done after every use.

Client preparation

It is important to be professional and communicate in a positive way at all times with your clients, models and colleagues. Further information on communication and behaviour can be found in *Presenting a professional image in a salon*.

Welcome the client or model and introduce yourself so that they feel at ease and start to feel confidence in you. Ask them to take a seat while you go through a few questions for your records. Record your client's details on their record card.

Visual inspection

Before starting any nail art designs, it is important to chat to the client and ask if they have any problems with the nails and surrounding skin. Also, ask if they are allergic to any products. While you are chatting about this, look at their hands and nails. Check if you can see anything that may prevent you from being able to carry out the nail art design (such as redness, flaking, swelling or soreness, or lifting of the nail plate).

Client comfort

When you have completed the visual study, position the client on a chair, making sure they are comfortable.

Drape a gown or towel across the client's lap to protect their clothing. A gown is also useful to protect the sleeves. If this isn't available tuck some tissue into the ends of the sleeves.

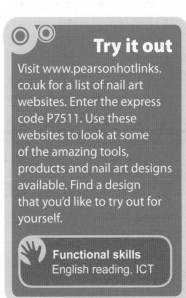

Try it out

Visit www.pearsonhotlinks.co.uk for a list of nail art websites. Enter the express code P7511. Use these websites to look at some of the amazing tools, products and nail art designs available. Find a design that you'd like to try out for yourself.

Functional skills
English reading, ICT

Just checking

1 What will you look for when carrying out a visual study of the client's nails and surrounding skin?

Design a 2D nail art image and adapt to a 3D surface

In this topic you will learn about:

- Designing 2D images and adapting these to a 3D surface

How do you think artists plan their paintings and designs? Find out about different ways that you can plan your nail art designs.

If you don't plan and organise carefully from the start, your design may not look the way you or your client had planned it to.

You will need to design a 2D image and then recreate it onto a 3D surface (such as an artificial or natural nail). You will need patience and a steady hand. This will be rewarded when you have created a design that is a piece of art.

Take photographs of each of step. In this way, you will have a record of how to do things next time. It is always good to be able to look back at photographs of completed designs.

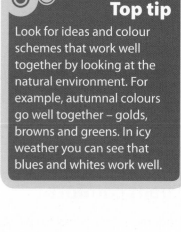

Top tip

Look for ideas and colour schemes that work well together by looking at the natural environment. For example, autumnal colours go well together – golds, browns and greens. In icy weather you can see that blues and whites work well.

Types of images

There are many different images that you can create. Here are just a few examples.

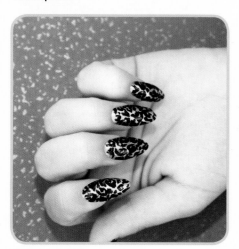

Animal design

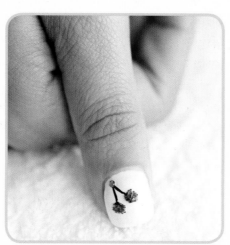

Glitter design

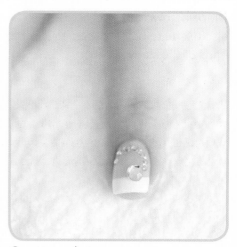

Gemstone design

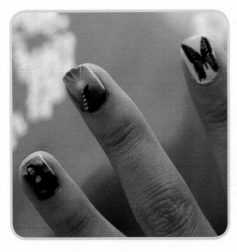

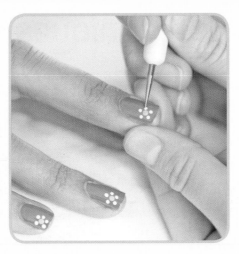

Transfer designs

Dotting tool design

Designing your 2D image

You are demonstrating your personality as well as your artistry when you design a 2D image that you feel confident you can adapt onto a 3D surface. Explore different designs and images to get ideas for your nail art design.

Explore designs from a range of places such as:
- celebrity magazines
- Internet images that you can print off
- science and nature books
- art and design images
- photographs.

Planning your design

Planning is important to the success of nail art design. Look at the image as a whole and then break it down into small easy steps. These steps will build up to the finished design.

The first thing you will always do is prepare the nails by wiping over them with non-acetone varnish remover. This makes sure the nail plate is clean and grease free.

Practise with simple designs at first. When you get more skilled you can try out different techniques. You must be able to complete your design in the time that you have. You must also make sure you have all the skills, tools, equipment and products that the design will need.

Carry out nail art techniques (1)

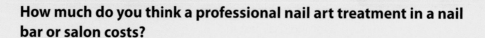

In this topic you will learn about:

- Carrying out nail art designs
- Aftercare advice

Q How much do you think a professional nail art treatment in a nail bar or salon costs?

Nail art design is a chance for people to express their personality – this goes for both the client and the person carrying out the nail art.

Take the time to see what fantastic designs are currently being applied to celebrity and fashion fingernails. Then it's your turn to create something spectacular or simple and effective.

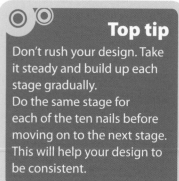

Top tip

Don't rush your design. Take it steady and build up each stage gradually.
Do the same stage for each of the ten nails before moving on to the next stage. This will help your design to be consistent.

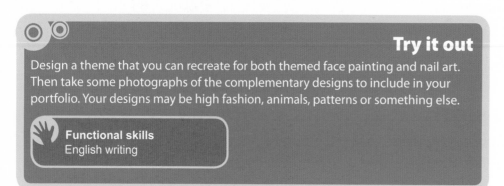

Try it out

Design a theme that you can recreate for both themed face painting and nail art. Then take some photographs of the complementary designs to include in your portfolio. Your designs may be high fashion, animals, patterns or something else.

Functional skills
English writing

There are many different techniques used to create nail art designs. On the following pages you will learn more about these techniques:
- Dotting
- French painting
- Marbling
- Colour blending

Simple use of a dotting tool

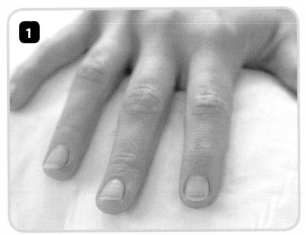

Paint the nails with a base coat

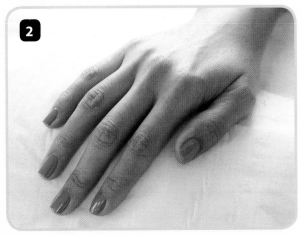

Paint the nails with your chosen colour

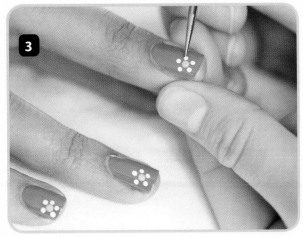

Use the large end of the dotting tool to create the centre of the daisy by applying a large dot to the nail with yellow acrylic nail paint. Then use the small end of the dotting tool to create white petals around the centre of the large dot

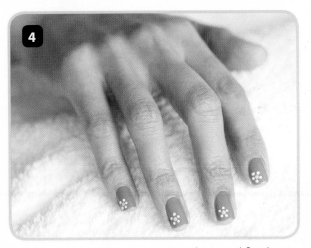

Apply protective top coat to give shine and finish to the nail art design

Aftercare advice

Advice you can give the client includes:

- Apply a coat of top coat every other day to prolong the life of the nail art design.
- Don't pick at any peeling colours. Stick it down temporarily with top coat by painting over a layer.
- Designs will last anything from a few days to two weeks. After this time you will need to remove them with non-acetone remover.

Just checking

1 List two points of aftercare advice.

2 Why is it best to do the same stage on each fingernail before moving on to the next stage?

Carry out nail art techniques (2)

Step-by-step funky French design

For this you will need base and top coats, green and pink glitter varnishes, white and black varnish and rhinestones.

1

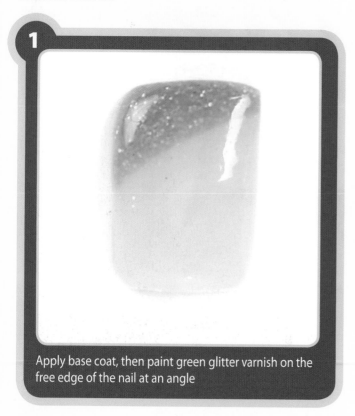

Apply base coat, then paint green glitter varnish on the free edge of the nail at an angle

2

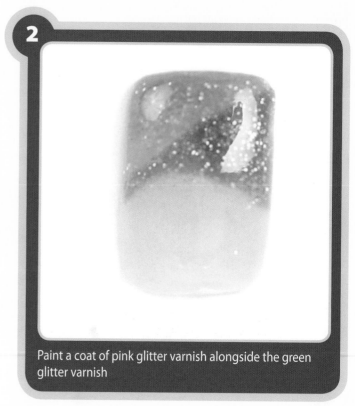

Paint a coat of pink glitter varnish alongside the green glitter varnish

3

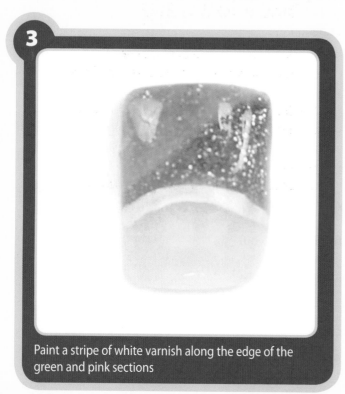

Paint a stripe of white varnish along the edge of the green and pink sections

4

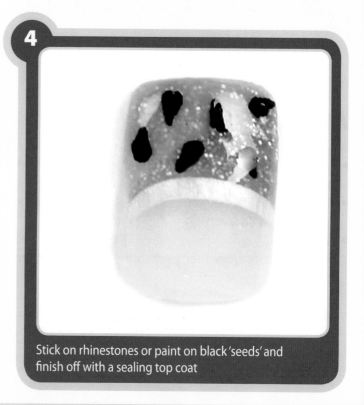

Stick on rhinestones or paint on black 'seeds' and finish off with a sealing top coat

Step-by-step marbling effect using dotting tools

1

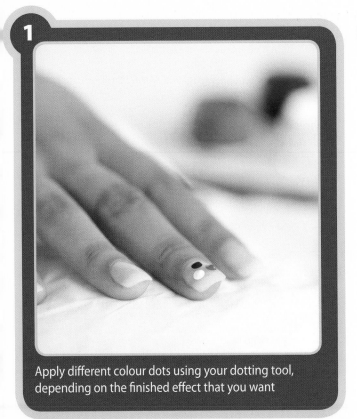

Apply different colour dots using your dotting tool, depending on the finished effect that you want

2

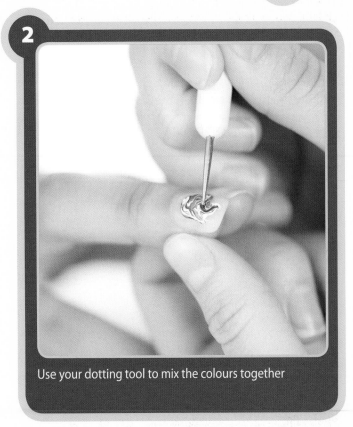

Use your dotting tool to mix the colours together

3

Continue to use your dotting tool, swirling the colours together until you have the marbling effect you are happy with

Colour blending

This technique is where you fade one colour into the next without having a definite line.

- First apply your base coat followed by the first colour.
- Then just before it dries, put on the second colour on the tip of your nails.
- You can do this again with a third coat if necessary.
- Wait until it dries off and put on a top coat.

Mapping grid

Unit	City & Guilds	VTCT	Edexcel	ITEC
Introduction to the hair and beauty sector	Unit 001 / Unit 101	Unit UV 30330/ Unit UV10343	Unit 1 / Unit 8	Unit 300 / Unit 313
Follow health and safety in the salon	Unit 113	-	-	-
Presenting a professional image in a salon	Unit 002 / Unit 102	Unit UV30331 / UV10344	Unit 2 / Unit 9	Unit 301 / Unit 314
Salon reception duties	Unit 114	-	-	-
Create an image using colour	Unit 005	Unit UV30334	Unit 7	Unit 304
Anatomy and physiology	The underpinning anatomy and physiology knowledge for all practical units is covered in a dedicated section.			
Shampoo and conditioning	Unit 003	Unit UV30336	Unit 5	Unit 305
Styling women's and men's hair	Unit 103 / Unit 104	Unit UV30337 / Unit UV30338	Unit 13 / Unit 14	Unit 311 / Unit 312
Plaiting and twisting hair	Unit 004 / Unit 105	Unit UV30341 / Unit UV30342	Unit 6 / Unit 15	Unit 306 / Unit 307
The art of dressing hair	Unit 215	Unit UV10345	Unit 17	
Skin care	Unit 006	Unit UV30335	Unit 3	Unit 302
Hand and foot care	Unit 007 / Unit 109 / Unit 110	Unit UV30332 /	Unit 4	Unit 303
Basic make-up application	Unit 106	Unit UV30339	Unit 10	Unit 310
Themed face painting	Unit 107	Unit UV30340	Unit 12	Unit 309
Nail art application	Unit 108	Unit UV30333	Unit 11	Unit 308

Answers to 'Just checking'

Introduction to the hair and beauty sector

Career opportunities and working patterns in the beauty sector, pp.10–11
1 Yes
2 www.habia.org
3 If you work full-time you will be expected to work for a minimum of 35 hours or even as many as 44. If you work part-time then you may work anything from just a few hours up to 35.

Career opportunities and working patterns in the hairdressing sector, pp.12–13
1 Yes
2 No

Different types of salon and the main hairdressing services and beauty treatments available, pp.14-15
1 Yes. They offer complementary services. There are lots of successful examples.
2 a Hair salon
  b Beauty salon
  c Hair salon
  d Beauty salon

Follow health and safety in the salon

Hazards and risks and the Health and Safety at Work Act, pp.18–19
1 c
2 c

More on hazards and risks, pp.20–21
1 True
2 False

COSHH, pp.22–23
1 Poisonous or flammable chemicals should be kept in a secure store when they are not being used.
2 Some examples include perm lotion, eyelash and eyebrow tint, relaxers, hair colourant, hydrogen peroxide and nail varnish remover.

PPE and the Electricity at Work Regulations, pp.24–25
1 c
2 b

Good posture and safe handling, pp.26–27
1 c
2 a

Sterilising equipment, pp.28–29
1 a
2 a

Emergencies and first aid, pp.30–31
1 c
2 c

Fire safety and fire extinguishers, pp.32–33
1 a

Presenting a professional image in a salon

Present a professional image, pp.36–37
1 Professional image means looking clean, tidy and presentable (both you and the salon).
2 a, c

How to maintain personal hygiene, pp.38–39
1 c
2 You are responsible for your personal hygiene.
3 Brush your teeth regularly and use breath freshener mints or spray after food.

Good communication in the salon, pp.40–41
1 a
2 If clients feel welcomed and looked after, the salon's professional image will be enhanced and business will improve through word of mouth.

Acting professionally in the salon, pp.42–43
1 a
2 b

Salon reception duties

Carrying out salon reception duties, pp.46–47
1 a
2 a, b

Recording salon appointments (1), pp.48–49
1 a, c
2 c

Recording salon appointments (2), pp.50–51
1 Written appointment book and computerised appointment system
2 'Appropriate appointment spacing' means the time differences between the clients booked into the salon for their service or treatment.

Create an image using colour

Knowing the colour spectrum, pp.54–55
1 a, c
2 b, d
3 d

Using the colour spectrum, pp.56–57
1 a, c
2 b

Anatomy and physiology

Hair structure and head and face shapes, pp.60–61
1 b
2 c

Hair features, pp.62–63
1 a
2 c

Hair growth patterns, pp.64–65
1 a
2 c

Hair types and the hair growth cycle, pp.66–67
1 b
2 c

Hairdressing – contra-indications, pp.68–69
1 b
2 d

The structure and functions of skin, pp.70–71
1 Five
2 Dermis

Skin types and conditions, pp.72–73
1 Normal, oily, dry, combination
2 Caucasian, Oriental, Asian, African-Caribbean

Skull and facial bones, pp.74–75
1 c
2 c
3 Any from:
  • The skull bones keep the muscles in place and protect the brain.
  • The bones of the face also protect the soft tissues inside the head.
  • Bone shapes our face and head.

The nails, pp.76–77
1 The grooves at the side of the nail guide the direction of the nail growth. The grooves also help to stop germs getting into the nail bed.
2 The nail plate is made up of layers of fat, moisture and growth cells.

Contra-indications for a facial treatment, pp.78–79
1 b
2 b

Contra-indications for a manicure/pedicure, pp.80–81
1 a
2 b

Shampoo and conditioning

Preparing for shampooing and conditioning, pp.84–85
1 c
2 d

Carry out the shampooing service, pp.86–87
1 a
2 c

Carry out the conditioning service, pp.88–89
1 Effleurage and petrissage
2 It's important to wrap and towel dry the client's hair before you move them to the workstation so they are comfortable and to stop the hair dripping.
3 The basin area should be left clean and tidy so that it's ready for the next client.

Styling women's and men's hair

Products, pp.92–93
1 c

Tools and equipment, pp.94–95
1 Pin tail comb
2 Round brush

Prepare for styling men's and women's hair, pp.96–97
1 The client should be properly gowned.

Techniques for styling women's and men's hair (1), pp.98–99
1 The airflow of the dryer should be directed from root to point.

Techniques for styling women's and men's hair (2), pp.100–101
1 You can control the hair by backcombing it and by working in small, controllable sections.

Setting the hair, pp.102–103
1 Big hair, bouncy curls, tight curls, etc.
2 The same size as the roller

Drying, dressing and pin-curling the hair, pp.104–105
1 You should let the hair cool down because a) the hair often feels dry when it's hot but, once it has cooled down, it may still be damp and b) it allows the hair to 'set' properly in its new shape.
2 To remove roller lines

Plaiting and twisting hair

Prepare for hair plaiting and twisting, pp.108–109
1 In case you can see anything that might cause a problem, for example, signs of traction alopecia.

Selecting products, tools and equipment for basic plaiting and twisting, pp.110–111
1 b

Introduction to carrying out plaiting and twisting techniques, pp.112–113
1 On scalp fit snugly to the head and off scalp are plaited along the length of the hair and secured at the ends.
2 Twists involve twisting the hair into sections either on or off the scalp. Plaits are sectioned into three or more sections and braided over each other.

Carrying out plaiting techniques, pp.114–115
1 a
2 c

Carrying out twisting techniques, pp.116–117
1 b
2 b

The art of dressing hair

Consult with client and evaluate the hair, pp.120–121
1 c
2 b

Styling products, pp.122–123
1 The two types are styling products and finishing products.
2 If serum is applied to fine hair it will weigh it down and make styling difficult.

Styling tools and equipment, pp.124–125
1 The correct way to clean a hand-held dryer is to unplug the dryer and wipe over with an alcohol-based wipe. The vent at the back should also be cleaned and then put back on.
2 You check that hair accessories are secure in a client's hair by asking them to move their head around.

Introduction to dressing hair, pp.126–127
1 a, c and d
2 b and c

Long hair looks – vertical roll and scalp plait, pp.128–129
1 b
2 c

Long hair looks – twists, backcombing and back brushing, pp.130–131
1 b and d
2 The cuticle is affected during backcombing.
3 d

Blow-drying, pp.132–133
1 When blow-drying, you should direct the airflow from root to point.
2 To make sure the heat is evenly spread, the hair is dried thoroughly and the section fits over the brush.

Styling and dressing hair (1), pp.134–135
1 You would use a diffuser to dry curly hair.
2 a
3 c

Styling and dressing hair (2), pp.136–137
1 You would use a clock spring pin curl to achieve tight curls in the nape.
2 So the new shape will stay in the hair for longer.

Carry out styling and dressing hair (3), pp.138–139
1 d
2 b

Structural hair changes and the effects of humidity, pp.140–141
1 b

Aftercare, pp.142–143
1 c

Skin care

Products, tools and equipment for skin care, pp.146–147
1 c
2 You can contaminate a pot or tub of cream by putting your fingers in it (instead of using a spatula).
3 Cream cleanser is best for mature skin.

Prepare for skin care, pp.148–149
1 Any two from: a) if you don't wash your hands before carrying out a treatment; b) if you use your fingers to scoop out cream from a tub or pot; c) if you blow your nose and don't wash your hands after; d) by using dirty tools
2 It is important to carry out a visual study of a client's skin to a) find out what their skin type is and b) to see if there are any contra-indications.
3 The four main skin types are normal, dry, oily and combination.

Carry out skin care, pp.150–151
1 The atmosphere should be calm, warm and confidential with soft lighting and relaxing music.
2 Support the client's neck by using a pillow or rolled-up towel.

Hand and foot care

Products for hand and foot care treatments, pp.156–157
1 Cuticle cream is used to soften and nourish the cuticles. It helps to prevent the skin splitting or drying out and makes it easier to gently push back the cuticles during treatment.
2 Buffing paste helps to smooth out the surface of the nail plate and add natural shine.

Equipment for hand and foot care treatments, pp.158–159
1 Orange wood sticks are used to apply cuticle cream to the cuticles and to push back the cuticles.
2 A manicure/finger bowl is a specially shaped gripper bowl with a lid that has a small hole in it for the thumb and a larger hole for the rest of the fingers.

Preparation for hand and foot care, pp.160–161
1 If you look the part you are more likely to feel confident and professional.
2 Any two from: nail varnish colour; contra-indications or disorders of the nail; nail and skin condition and nail shape

Nail shapes and nail structure, pp.162–163
1 Any three from: oval; round; square; pointed
2 Toenails are best naturally square, not shaped and cut straight across.
3 Pointed.

Factors that could influence treatment, pp.164–165
1 You are looking for any condition that might mean you cannot carry out the treatment or that requires you to adapt it. For example, bruising or cuts, severe nail separation or signs of allergy.
2 When you carry out a manual check of the client's nails and surrounding skin you are looking to see if:
 • the skin is soft and smooth, or dry and flaky
 • the nails are smooth or if they have ridges
 • the cuticles are rough or smooth.

Contra-indications and contra-actions, pp.166–167
1 A contra-indication is a condition that may prevent or restrict treatment.
2 A contra-action is an unwanted condition that may happen during or after a treatment.

Carry out hand and foot care treatments, pp.168–169
1 Three pieces of aftercare advice you could give include:
 • Don't pick at nails and cuticles.
 • Use hand cream or moisturiser daily.
 • Have regular manicures and pedicures.
2 Hand and foot massage softens the skin, relaxes the muscles and improves the circulation.

Basic make-up application

Equipment for make-up, pp.176–177
1 If you scoop out cream from pots using your fingers, you could contaminate the cream with bacteria, which would then spread to other clients.
2 You should split the tissues before use because it is more economical. It's also easier to blot with them when have been split.

Tools for make-up, pp.178–179
1 Any three from: blusher; eyeshadow; sponge applicator; lip brush; eyeliner brush; brow brush
2 Disposable make-up brushes are used to prevent cross-infection.

Products for make-up (1), pp.180–181
1 Before moisturiser, after cleanser
2 10 minutes

Products for make-up (2), pp.182–183
1 Concealer is used to cover up spots and blemishes.

2 Foundation should be applied with a make-up sponge.

Factors influencing make-up 1, pp.184–185
1 A cream
2 The four basic face shapes are round, oval, square and oblong.

Factors influencing make-up (2), pp.186–187
1 Natural daylight
2 It makes make-up colours look colder.
3 Liquid eyeliner and false lashes

Prepare for make-up, pp.188–189
1 Look for any signs of redness or inflammation that could be a sign of a contra-indication.
2 Any four from: personal client contact details; contra-indications or disorders of the skin and/or eyes; skin condition and skin type; make-up products and techniques used; your name; date of treatment; client signature
3 Wash brushes in warm, soapy water and leave to air dry. This must be done after every client. Or you could use disposable brushes and sponges.

Applying basic make-up, pp.190–191
1 Lip liner is used to improve the shape of the lips and prevent colour spreading out.
2 Powder is used to set foundation.

Applying and removing basic make-up, pp.192–193
1 A sponge applicator is best for applying eyeshadow.
2 Tell the client to remove their make-up thoroughly and not to keep touching their face.

Themed face painting

Face painting products, pp.196–197
1 The two types of glitter are loose and in gel form.
2 Face paints should be non-toxic and water-based to prevent allergies and so they are easy to remove with water.

Tools and equipment for face painting, pp.198–199
1 Any three from: fine flat face painting brush; fine round face painting brush; large flat face painting brush; medium flat face painting brush; medium round multi-purpose painting brush
2 The two types of face painting sponges are a latex sponge and a stipple sponge.

Factors influencing themed face painting, pp.200–201
1 Any three from: client age; size and shape of face; skin colour and type; theme or occasion
2 Typical designs that a young child might ask for are cartoon characters or animals.

Prepare for themed face painting, pp.202–203
1 If you are carrying out face painting on a child you should be professional, well behaved and patient.
2 Before carrying out face painting on a child under 16 you must first get parental consent.

Design a 3D image from a 2D image, pp.204–205
1 You should remove water-based face paints with cleansing wipes, water or cleanser.
2 You should remove glitter and glitter gels with a thick cleansing cream.

Nail art

Products for nail art, pp.210–211
1 Nail varnish remover that contains acetone can dissolve nail structures.
2 Glitter varnish and glitter dust

Tools and equipment for nail art, pp.212–213
1 Stripes created by the fan brush are more like an airbrushing effect.
2 Any three from: striping brush; fan brush; orange wood stick; multi-purpose scissors; cotton buds; card

Factors influencing nail art design, pp.214–215
1 Any three from: fashion; pricing; time; nail shape; length
2 Neutral colours would be best for someone with blue tones to their skin.

Prepare for nail art design, pp.216–217
1 When carrying out a visual study of the client's nails and surrounding skin you should look for redness, swelling, soreness, lifting of the nail plate or flaking.

Design a 2D nail art image and adapt to a 3D surface, pp.218–219
1 Prepare the nail before painting it by degreasing it with nail varnish remover.
2 Any two from: science and nature books; photographs; celebrity magazines

Carry out nail art techniques (1), pp.220–222
1 Two points of aftercare advice include:
 • Don't peel off flaking designs.
 • Apply a top coat every other day to prolong the life of the design.
2 It is best to do the same stage on each fingernail before moving on to the next stage so that your design is consistent.

Index

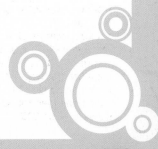